Clinical Skills

e of the conditions se

ROGER BLACKWOOD

MA, FRCP
Consultant Physician, Wexham Park Hospital, Slough,
and Honorary Consultant Physician at
Hammersmith Hospital, London

CHRIS HATTON

FRCP, FRCPath
Consultant Haematologist,
Department of Haematology,
The John Radcliffe Hospital

Fourth edition

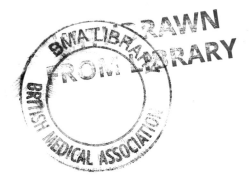

Blackwell
Science

© 1993, 1991, 1997, 2003 by Blackwell Science Ltd
a Blackwell Publishing Company
Blackwell Science, Inc., 350 Main Street, Malden, MA 02148-5018, USA
Blackwell Science Ltd, Osney Mead, Oxford OX2 0EL, UK
Blackwell Science Asia Pty, 54 University Street, Carlton South, Victoria 3053, Australia
Blackwell Wissenschafts Verlag, Kurfürstendamm 57, 10707 Berlin, Germany

The right of the Authors to be identified as the Authors of this Work has been asserted in accordance with the Copyright, Designs and Patents Act 1988.

First published (under Lecture notes on clinical skills and Examination) 1983
Second edition 1991
Four Dragons edition 1991
Third edition 1997
International edition 1997
Reprinted 1998 (twice), 2000
Fourth edition 2003

Library of Congress Cataloging-in-Publication Data

Blackwood, Roger.
   Lecture notes on clinical skills/
   Roger Blackwood.
      p.   cm.
   Rev. ed. of: Lecture notes on clinical skills/
   Robert Turner, Roger Blackwood, 3rd ed. 1997.
   Includes index.
   ISBN 0-632-06511-7
   1. Medical history taking—Handbooks, manuals, etc.
   2. Physical diagnosis—Handbooks, manuals, etc.
   [DNLM: 1. Medical History Taking—Handbooks.
   2. Physical Examination—Handbooks. WB 39 B632L 2002]
   I. Hatton, Chris. II. Turner, Robert (Robert Charles), 1938–
   Lecture notes on clinical skills. III. Title.
   RC65. T87 2002
   616.07 5—dc21

ISBN 0-632-06511-7

A catalogue record for this title is available from the British Library

Set in 9/11 $^1\!/_2$ Gill Sans by SNP Best-set Typesetter Ltd, Hong Kong
Printed and bound in the UK by MPG Books Ltd, Bodmin, Cornwall

For further information on Blackwell Science, visit our website:
http://www.blackwellpublishing.com

Contents

Preface

When a medical student first approaches a patient, he has to:
- O *develop a suitable doctor–patient relationship*
- O *master many relevant skills and techniques*
- O *develop an enquiring and intelligent approach*

These notes are intended to assist with all these aspects. They particularly aim to inform the reader succinctly at each stage:
- O *what you should do*
- O *how you should think*

Although the notes could be simply used as a manual, it is hoped that the student will quickly learn the art of altering his approach, according to the specific manifestations of illness and the personality of the patient.

It is intended that the book be easily pocketed, and that it could be read near the bedside. In general the pages are arranged with simple instructions on the left, with important aspects requiring action marked with an open dot (O). Subsidiary lists are marked with a dash (–). On the right are brief details of clinical situations and diseases which are relevant to abnormal findings.

The notes have been used in the Oxford Clinical Medical School for 20 years. We much appreciate the invaluable guidance and comments we have received from many colleagues and students. Different doctors use slightly different techniques in taking a history and examination, and inevitably some would prefer slightly different instructions.

Throughout the text the pronoun he is used to refer to doctors, students and patients. This is not intended to imply that all doctors, students and patients are male and we hope the reader is not offended by what has been adopted as an economical linguistic convention.

In this new edition we have updated the text in many of the chapters. We are particularly grateful to Dr Briley for helping us with the neurology chapter. With the help of friends and colleagues we have added some basic haematology and biochemistry which we hope will be useful to the clinical student and junior doctor. Remember, the most important clinical skill is to take a good history and perform a careful examination.

Chris Hatton
Roger Blackwood
Oxford 2002

Acknowledgements

We are grateful to many colleagues and students who have made suggestions. The book has benefited from their suggestions, but any faults or omissions are those of the authors. Specific advice was received from:

History	Bill Rosenberg, Tony Hope
Skin	Terence Ryan, Sue Burge
Eyes	Peggy Frith
Orthopaedics	Roger Smith, Chris Bulstrode
Surgery	Jack Collins, Michael Greenall
Heart	Oliver Ormerod
Lungs	Donald Lane
Gastroenterology	Derek Jewell
Mental state	Michael Sharpe
Neurology	Michael Donaghy, Robin Kennett, Dennis Briley
Disability	Simon Winner, Sebastian Fairweather
Imaging	Niall Moore, David Lindsell, Wattie Fletcher, Andy Molyneux, Basil Shepstone
Evidence-based medicine	David Sackett
Therapies	Chris Garrard, Lucy Belson, Ben Aszali
Biochemistry and endocrinology	Jonathan Kay, Nicki Metson, Louise Bowman
History and examination	Becky Rippon

The visual acuity reading charts (Appendices 1 and 2) are reproduced courtesy of Keeler Ltd; and the cardiac arrest instructions (Appendix 5) are redrawn courtesy of the European Resuscitation Council (© 1994).

The colour plates are reproduced courtesy of Department of Medical Illustration, Heatherwood and Wexham Park Hospitals Trust (Plates 1a–d, 2d, 2f, 3a, 3c–e, 4b, 5b–f, 6a, 6c–f), King Edward VII Hospital, Windsor (Plates 1e, 1f, 2a, 2b, 4a, 4c, 4e), Department of Medical Illustration, John Radcliffe Hospital, Oxford (Plates 2e, 4d, 5a, 6b), Department of Medical Illustration, Radcliffe Infirmary, Oxford (Plates 3f, 4f).

INTRODUCTION

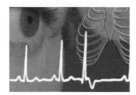

The First Approach

General principles

General objectives

When the student (or doctor) approaches a patient there are **four initial objectives**:

o **Obtain a professional rapport with the patient and gain his confidence.**

o **Obtain all relevant information which allows assessment of the illness, and provisional diagnoses.**

o **Obtain general information regarding the patient, his background, social situation and problems. In particular it is necessary to find out how the illness has affected him, his family, friends, colleagues and his life.**

> The assessment of the patient as a whole is of utmost importance.

o **Understand the patient's own ideas about his problems, his major concerns and what he expects from the hospital admission, outpatient or general practice consultation.**

> Remember medicine is just as much about worry as disease. Whatever the illness, whether chest infection or cancer, anxiety about what may happen is often uppermost in the patient's mind. **Listen attentively.**

The following notes provide a guide as to how one obtains the necessary information.

Specific objectives

In taking a history or making an examination there are **two complementary aims**:

o **Obtain all possible information about a patient and his illness (a database).**
o **Solve the problem as to the diagnoses.**

Analytical approach

For each symptom or sign one needs to think of a differential diagnosis, and of other relevant information (by history, examination or investigation) which one will need to support or refute these possible diagnoses. A good history combines these two facets, and one should never approach the patient with just a set series of rote questions. However, until one knows more medicine, one cannot know the possible significance of the information one gains, and the obvious change of questioning which this might entail. These notes provide background information enabling a full history and examination to be taken. This provides a necessary basis for a later, more inquisitive approach which should develop as knowledge about illnesses is acquired.

Self-reliance

The student must take his own history, make his own examination and write his own clinical records. After 1 month he should be sufficiently proficient that his notes could become the final hospital record. The student should add a summary including his assessment of the problem list, provisional diagnoses and preliminary investigations. Initially these will be incomplete and occasionally incorrect. Nevertheless, this exercise will help to inculcate an enquiring approach and to highlight areas in which further questioning, investigation or reading is needed.

What is important when you start?

At the basis of all medicine is clinical competence. No amount of knowledge will make up for poor technique.

Over the first few weeks it is essential to learn the **basic ABC of clinical medicine**, covered in these notes:

o **how to relate to patients**
o **how to take a good history efficiently, knowing which question to ask next and avoiding leading questions**

o **how to examine patients in a logical manner, in a set routine which will mean you will not miss an unexpected sign**

> You will be surprised how often students can fail an exam, not because of lack of knowledge but because they have not mastered elementary clinical skills. These notes are written to try and help you to identify what is important and to help relate findings to common clinical situations.

There is nothing inherently difficult about clinical medicine. You will quickly become clinically competent if you:

o **apply yourself**
o **initially learn by rote which skills are appropriate for each situation**

Common sense

Common sense is the cornerstone of medicine

o **Always be aware of the patient's needs.**
o **Always evaluate what important information is needed:**
  - **to obtain the diagnosis**
  - **to give appropriate therapy**
  - **to ensure continuity of care at home**

Many mistakes are made by being side-tracked by aspects that are not important.

Learning

Your clinical skills and knowledge can soon develop with good organization.

o **Take advantage of seeing many patients** in hospital, in clinics and in the community. It is particularly helpful to be present when patients are being admitted as emergencies or are being seen in a clinic for the first time.
o **Obtain a wide experience of clinical diseases,** how they affect patients and how they are managed.

> Medicine is a practical subject and first-hand experience is invaluable. The more patients you can clerk yourself, the sooner you will become proficient and the more you will learn about patients and their diseases.

Building up knowledge

At first medicine seems a huge subject and each fact you learn seems to be an isolated piece of information. How will you ever be able to learn what is required? You will find after a few months that the bits of information do interrelate and that you are able to put new bits of information into context. The pieces of the jigsaw puzzle begin to fit together and then your confidence will increase. Although you will need to learn many facts, it is equally important to acquire the attitude of questioning, reasoning and knowing when and where to go to seek additional information.

o **Choose a medium-sized student's textbook in which you read up about each disease you see or each problem you encounter.**

> **Attaching knowledge to individual patients is a great help in acquiring and remembering facts.** To practise medicine without a textbook is like a sailor without a chart, whereas to study books rather than patients is like a sailor who does not go to sea.

Understand the scientific background of disease, including the advances that are being made and how these could be applied to improve care.

o **Regularly pick up and read the editorials or any articles which interest you** in a general medical journal such as *New England Journal of Medicine*, *Lancet* or *British Medical Journal*.

> Even if at first you are not able to put information into context, they will keep you in touch with new developments that add interest. Nevertheless, it is not sensible to delve too deeply into any one subject when you are just beginning.

Relationships

Training to become a doctor includes the distinct challenges of learning:

o **to have a natural, sincere, receptive and, when necessary, supportive relationship with patients and staff**

o **the optimum means of working with patients and colleagues to facilitate good care**

Presentation of your findings and communication in general

Chapter 10 indicates how you should present patients on ward rounds or at meetings.

Ancillary investigations

Introductory information about several common clinical investigations is given in Chapter 11, together with a simple guide to reading an electrocardiogram (ECG) in Chapter 12.

Treatment of illness

You will soon witness various treatments being given. Chapter 15 details the essentials of common emergency therapies that you will encounter.

Evidence-based medicine, statistical analyses and interpretation of tests

Many advances in medicine are occurring. It is helpful to have the background knowledge to allow evaluation of new information, clinical trials and techniques. Chapter 13 provides overviews of interpretation of data.

Bon voyage

In training to become a doctor, you have:

o the privilege of developing supportive relationships with patients and staff
o the chance to develop special practical skills
o the opportunity to appreciate the academic developments that are being made

We wish you good luck with your career and the all-important mastering of basic clinical skills.

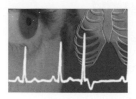

CHAPTER 1

History Taking

General procedures

Approaching the patient

- ○ Look the part of a doctor and put the patient at ease. Be confident and quietly friendly.
- ○ Greet the patient: 'Good morning, Mr Smith'.
- ○ Shake the patient's hand or place your hand on his if he is ill.
- ○ State your name and that you are a student doctor helping staff care for patients.
- ○ Make sure the patient is comfortable.
- ○ Explain that you wish to ask the patient questions to find out what happened to him.

> Inform the patient how long you are likely to take and what to expect. For example, after discussing what has happened to the patient, you would like to examine him.

Usual sequence of events

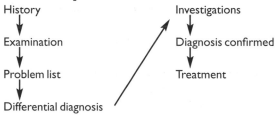

History
↓
Examination
↓
Problem list
↓
Differential diagnosis

Investigations
↓
Diagnosis confirmed
↓
Treatment

Importance of the history

It identifies:
- — what has happened
- — the personality of the patient
- — how the illness has affected him and his family
- — any specific anxieties
- — the physical and social environment
- — It establishes the physician–patient relationship.
- — It often gives the diagnosis.

O **Find the principal symptoms or symptom. Ask:**
- — **'What has the problem been?'**
- — **'What made you go to the doctor?'**

Avoid:
- — 'What's wrong?' or 'What brought you here?'

O **Let the patient tell his story in his own words as much as possible.**

At first listen and then take discreet notes as he talks.
When learning to take a history there can be a tendency to ask too many questions in the first 2 minutes. After asking the first question you should normally allow the patient to talk uninterrupted for up to 2 minutes.

Do not worry if the story is not entirely clear, or if you do not think the information being given is of diagnostic significance. If you interrupt too early, you run the risk of overlooking an important symptom or anxiety.

- — **You will be learning about what the patient thinks is important.**
- — **You have the opportunity to judge how you are going to proceed.**

Different patients give histories in very different ways. Some patients will need to be encouraged to enlarge on their answers to your questions; with other patients you may need to ask specific questions and to interrupt in order to prevent too rambling a history. Think consciously about the approach you will adopt. If you need to interrupt the patient, do so clearly and decisively.

○ **Try, if feasible, to conduct a conversation rather than an interrogation, following the patient's train of thoughts.**

> You will usually need to ask follow-up questions on the main symptoms to obtain a full understanding of what they were and of the chain of events.

○ **Obtain a full description of the patient's principal complaints.**

○ **Enquire about the sequence of symptoms and events.**

> Beware pseudomedical terms, e.g. 'gastric flu' — enquire what happened

○ **Do not ask leading questions.**

> A central aim in taking the history is to understand patients' symptoms from their own point of view. It is important not to tarnish the patient's history by your own expectations. For example, do not ask a patient whom you suspect might be thyrotoxic: 'Do you find hot weather uncomfortable?' This invites the answer 'Yes' and then a positive answer becomes of little diagnostic value. Ask the open question: 'Do you particularly dislike either hot or cold weather?'

○ **Be sensitive to a patient's mood and non-verbal responses.**

> e.g. hesitancy in revealing emotional content.

○ **Be understanding, receptive and matter-of-fact without excessive sympathy.**

○ **Rarely show surprise or reproach.**

○ **Clarify symptoms and obtain a problem list.**

When the patient has finished describing the symptom or symptoms:

— **briefly summarize the symptoms**

— **ask whether there are any other main problems**

> For example say 'You have mentioned two problems: pain on the left side of your tummy, and loose motions over the last 6 weeks. Before we talk about those in more detail, are there any other problems I should know about?'

Usual sequence of history

— nature of principal complaints, e.g. chest pain, poor home circumstances

- history of present complaint—details of current illness
- enquiry of other symptoms (see Functional enquiry, p. 10)
- **past history**
- **family history**
- **personal and social history**

o **If one's initial enquiries make it apparent that one section is of more importance than usual (e.g. previous relevant illnesses or operation), then relevant enquiries can be brought forward to an earlier stage in the history (e.g. past history after finding principal complaints).**

History of present illness

o **Start your written history with a single sentence** summing up what your patient is complaining of. It should be like the banner headline of a newspaper. For example:

c/o chest pain for 6 months

o **Determine the chronology of the illness by asking:**
- 'How and when did your illness begin?' or
- 'When did you first notice anything wrong?' or
- 'When did you last feel completely well?'

o **Begin by stating when the patient was last perfectly well.** Describe symptoms in **chronological order of onset.**

Both the **date of onset** and the **length of time** prior to admission should be recorded. Symptoms should never be dated by the day of the week as this later becomes meaningless.

o **Obtain a detailed description of each symptom by asking:**
- 'Tell me what the pain was like', for example. Make sure you ask about all symptoms, whether they seem relevant or not.

o **With all symptoms obtain the following details:**
- **duration**
- **onset—sudden or gradual**
- **what has happened since:**
  - **constant or periodic**
  - **frequency**
  - **getting worse or better**

- **precipitating or relieving factors**
- **associated symptoms**
○ **If pain is a symptom also determine the following:**
- **site**
- **radiation**
- **character**, e.g. ache, pressure, shooting, stabbing, dull
- **severity**, e.g. 'Did it interfere with what you were doing? Does it keep you awake?'
- have you ever had this pain before?
- is the pain associated with nausea, sweating, e.g. angina?

Avoid technical language when describing a patient's history. Do not say 'the patient complained of melaena', rather: 'the patient complained of passing loose, black, tarry motions'.

Supplementary history

When patients are unable to give an adequate or reliable history, the necessary information must be obtained from friends or relations. A history from a person who has witnessed a sudden event is often helpful.

Accordingly, the student should arrange with the houseman to be present when the relatives or witnesses are interviewed. This is particularly important with patients suffering from disease of the central nervous system. The date and source of such information should be written in the notes.

When necessary, arrange for an interpreter.

Make use of GP's letter and contact GP if necessary.

Functional enquiry

This is a checklist of symptoms not already discovered.

Do not ask questions already covered in establishing the principal symptoms. This list may detect other symptoms.

○ **Modify your questioning according to the nature of the suspected disease, available time and circumstances.**

If during the functional enquiry a positive answer is obtained, full details must be elicited. Asterisks (*) denote questions which must nearly always be asked.

General questions

O Ask about the following points:
- *Appetite: 'What is your appetite like? Do you feel like eating?'
- *Weight: 'Have you lost or gained weight recently?'
- *General well-being: 'Do you feel well in yourself?'
- Fatigue: 'Are you more or less tired than you used to be?'
- Fever or chills: 'Have you felt hot or cold? Have you shivered?'
- Night sweats: 'Have you noticed any sweating at night or any other time?'
- Aches or pains.
- Rash: 'Have you had any rash recently? Does it itch?'
- Lumps and bumps.

Cardiovascular and respiratory system

O Ask about the following points:
- *Chest pain: 'Have you recently had any pain or discomfort in the chest?'

   The most common causes of chest pain are:

   Ischaemic heart disease: severe constricting, central chest pain radiating to the neck, jaw and left arm. *Angina* is this pain precipitated by exercise or emotion; relieved by rest. In a *myocardial infarction* the pain may come on at rest, be more severe and last hours.

   Pleuritic pain: sharp, localized pain, usually lateral; worse on inspiration or cough.

   Anxiety or panic attacks are a very common cause of chest pain. Enquire about circumstances that bring on an attack.
- *Shortness of breath: 'Are you breathless at any time?'

   Breathlessness (*dyspnoea*) and chest pain must be accurately described. The degree of exercise which brings on the symptoms must be noted (e.g. climbing one flight of stairs, after 0.5 km (1/4 mile) walk).
- Shortness of breath on lying flat (*orthopnoea*): 'Do you get

breathless in bed? What do you do then? Does it get worse or better on sitting up? How many pillows do you use? Can you sleep without them?'

— **Waking up breathless**: 'Do you wake at night with any symptoms? Do you gasp for breath? What do you do then?'

> Orthopnoea (breathless when lying flat) and paroxysmal nocturnal dyspnoea (waking up breathless, relieved on sitting up) are features of left heart failure.

— ***Ankle swelling**.

> Common in congestive cardiac failure (right heart failure).

— **Palpitations**: 'Are you aware of your heart beating?'

> Palpitations may be:
> - single thumps (ectopics)
> - slow or fast
> - regular or irregular
>
> Ask the patient to tap them out.
>
> Paroxysmal tachycardia (sudden attacks of palpitations) usually starts and finishes abruptly.

— ***Cough**: 'Do you have a cough? Is it a dry cough or do you cough up sputum? When do you cough?'

— **Sputum**: 'What colour is your sputum? How much do you cough up?'

> Green sputum usually indicates an acute chest infection. Clear sputum daily during winter months suggests chronic bronchitis. Frothy sputum suggests left heart failure.

— ***Blood in sputum** (haemoptysis): 'Have you coughed up blood?'

> Haemoptysis must be taken very seriously. Causes include:
> carcinoma of bronchus
> pulmonary embolism
> mitral stenosis
> tuberculosis
> bronchiectasis

— **Black-outs** (syncope): 'Have you had any black-outs or faints? Did you feel light-headed or did the room go round? Did you lose consciousness? Did you have any warning? Can you remember what happened?'

— ***Smoking**: 'Do you smoke? How many cigarettes do you smoke?'

Gastrointestinal system

O Ask about the following points:

— **Mouth ulcers**

— **Nausea**: 'Are there times when you feel sick?'

— **Vomiting**: 'Do you vomit? What is it like?'

> 'Coffee grounds' vomit suggests altered blood.
>
> Old food suggests *pyloric stenosis*.
>
> If blood what colour is it—dark or bright red?

— **Difficulty in swallowing** (*dysphagia*): 'Do you have difficulty swallowing? Where does it stick?'

> For solids: often organic obstruction.
>
> For fluids: often neurological or psychological.

— **Indigestion**: 'Do you have any discomfort in your stomach after eating?'

— **Abdominal pain**: 'Where is the pain? How is it connected to meals or opening your bowels? What relieves the pain?'

— ***Bowel habit**: 'Is your bowel habit regular? How many times do you open your bowels per day? Do you have to open your bowels at night?' (*often a sign of true pathology*).

> If *diarrhoea* is suggested, the number of motions per day and their nature (blood? pus? mucus?) must be established.
>
> 'What are your motions like?' The stools may be pale, bulky and float (fat in stool—*steatorrhoea*) or tarry from digested blood (*melaena*—usually from upper gastrointestinal tract).
>
> Bright blood on the surface of a motion may be from *haemorrhoids*, whereas blood in a stool may signify *cancer* or *inflammatory bowel disease*.

— **Jaundice**: 'Is your urine dark? Are your stools pale? What tablets have you been taking recently? Have you had any recent injections or transfusions? Have you been abroad recently? How much alcohol do you drink?'

> Jaundice may be:

- **obstructive** (dark urine pale stools) from:
  carcinoma of the head of the pancreas gallstones
- **hepatocellular** (dark urine, pale stools may develop) from:
  ethanol (*cirrhosis*)
  drugs or transfusions (*viral hepatitis*)
  drug reactions or infections (travel abroad, *viral hepatitis* or *amoebae*)
- **haemolytic** (unconjugated bilirubin is bound to albumin and is not secreted in the urine)

Genitourinary system

O Ask about the following points:
- **Dysuria**: pain on passing urine usually burning (*often a sign of infection*).
- **Loin pain**: 'Any pain in your back?'
  Pain in the loins suggests pyelonephritis.
- ***Urine**: 'Are your waterworks all right? Do you pass a lot of water at night? Do you have any difficulty passing water? Is there blood in your water?' —*haematuria*.
  Polyuria and *nocturia* occur in *diabetes*.
  Prostatism results in slow onset of urination, a poor stream and terminal dribbling.
- **Sex**: 'Any problems with intercourse or making love?'
- ***Menstruation**: 'Any problems with your periods? Do you bleed heavily? Do you bleed between periods?'
  Vaginal bleeding between periods or after the menopause raises the possibility of *cervical* or *uterine cancer*.
- **Vaginal discharge**.
- **Menstrual cycle**: last menstrual period (LMP) and abormal vaginal bleeding:
  inter-menstrual bleeding
  post-menopausal bleeding
  post-coital bleeding
- **Pain on intercourse** (*dyspareunia*) and whether this is superficial or deep.

Nervous system

o Ask about the following points:

  — ***Headache**: 'Do you have any headaches? Where are they, when do you get headaches?'

> e.g. *early morning headaches may suggest raised intracranial pressure — tumour.*
>
> Are the headaches associated with flashing lights (*amaurosis fugax*).

  — **Vision**: 'Do you have any blurred or double vision?'

  — **Hearing**: ask about tinnitus, deafness and exposure to noise.

  — **Dizziness**: 'Do you have any dizziness or episodes when the world goes round (*vertigo*)?'

> Dizziness with light-headed symptoms, when sudden in onset, may be *cardiac* (enquire about palpitations). When slow, onset may be *vasovagal* 'fainting' or an *internal haemorrhage.*
>
> Vertigo may be from *ear disease* (enquire about deafness, earache or discharge) or *brainstem dysfunction.*

  — **Unsteady gait**: 'Any difficulty walking or running?'

  — **Weakness**.

  — **Numbness** or increased sensation: 'Any patches of numbness?'

  — **Pins and needles**.

  — **Sphincter disturbance**: 'Any difficulties holding your water/bowels?' (*a very important sign of spinal cord compression*).

  — **Fits or faints**: 'Have you had any funny episodes?'

> The following details should be sought from the patient and any observer:
>
>   — **duration**
>   — **frequency** and length of attacks
>   — **time of attacks**, e.g. if standing, at night
>   — **mode of onset and termination**
>   — **premonition or aura**, light-headed or vertigo
>   — **biting of tongue, loss of sphincter control, injury, etc.**
>
> *Grand mal epilepsy* classically produces sudden unconsciousness without any warning and on waking the patient

feels drowsy with a headache, sore tongue, and has been incontinent.

Mental state

o Ask about the following points:
  - **Depression**: 'How is your mood? Happy or sad? If depressed, how bad? Have you lost interest in things? Can you still enjoy things? How do you feel about the future?'

    'Has anything happened in your life to make you depressed? Do you feel guilty about anything?'

    If the patient appears depressed: 'Have you ever thought of suicide? How long have you felt like this? Is there a specific problem? Have you felt like this before?'
  - **Active periods**: 'Do you have periods in which you are particularly active?'

    Susceptibility to depression may be a personality trait. In *bipolar depression*, swings to *mania* (excess activity, rapid speech and excitable mood) can recur. Enquire about interest, concentration, irritability, sleep difficulties.
  - **Anxiety**: 'Have you worried a lot recently? Do you get anxious? In what situations? Are there any situations you avoid because you feel anxious?'

    'Do you worry about your health? Any worries in your job or with your family? Any financial worries?'

    'Do you have panic attacks? What happens?'
  - **Sleep**: 'Any difficulties sleeping? Do you have difficulty getting to sleep? Do you wake early?'

    Difficulties of sleep are commonly associated with depression or anxiety.

A more complete assessment of mental state is given in Chapter 6.

The eye

o Ask about the following points:
  - **Eye pain, photophobia or redness**: 'Have the eyes been red, uncomfortable or painful?'

— Painful red eye, particularly with photophobia may be serious and due to:

  iritis (ankylosing spondylitis, Reiter's disease, sarcoid, Behçet's disease)

  scleritis (systemic vasculitis)

  corneal ulcer

  acute glaucoma

  photophobia may be a sign of meningitis

— Painless red eye may be:

  episcleritis

  temporary and of no consequence

  systemic vasculitis

— Sticky red eye may be *conjunctivitis* (usually infective).

— Itchy eye may be *allergic*, e.g. *hayfever*.

— Gritty eye may be dry (sicca or *Sjögren's syndrome*).

— **Clarity of vision**: 'Has your vision been blurred?'

  — Blurring of vision for either near or distance alone may be an error of focus, helped by spectacles.

  — Loss of central vision (or of top or bottom half) in one eye may be due to a *retinal or optic nerve disorder*.

  — Transient complete blindness in one eye lasting for minutes — *amaurosis fugax* (fleeting blindness):

    suggests retinal arterial blockage from embolus may be from *carotid atheroma* (listen for bruit) may have a cardiac source

  — Subtle difficulties with vision, difficulty reading — problems at the chiasm, or visual path behind it:

    complete *bitemporal hemianopia — tumour* pressure on chiasm

    homonymous hemianopia: posterior cerebral or optic radiation lesion — usually *infarct or tumour;* rarely complains of 'half vision', but may have difficulty reading

— **Diplopia**: 'Have you ever seen double?'

  Diplopia may be due to:

  — *lesion* of the motor cranial nerves III, IV or VI

  — *third-nerve palsy*

    causes double vision in all directions

often with dilatation of the pupil and ptosis
the eye hangs 'down and out'
— *fourth-nerve palsy*
causes doubling looking down and in (as when reading)
with images separated horizontally and vertically and tilted
(not parallel)
— *sixth-nerve palsy*
causes horizontal, level and parallel doubling
worse on looking to the affected side
— *muscular disorder*
e.g. thyroid-related (see below)
myasthenia gravis (weakness after muscle use, antibodies to
nerve end-plates)

Locomotor system

○ Ask about the following points:

— **Pain, stiffness, or swelling of joints**: 'When and how did it start?
Have you injured the joint?'

There are innumerable causes of *arthritis* (painful, swollen,
tender joints) and *arthralgia* (painful joints). Patients may incorrectly attribute a problem to some injury.

Osteoarthritis is a joint 'wearing out', and is often asymmetric, involving weight-bearing joints such as the hip or knee.
Exercise makes the joint pain worse.

Rheumatoid arthritis is a generalized autoimmune disease
with symmetrical involvement. In the hands, fusiform swelling
of the interphalangeal joints is accompanied by swollen
metacarpophalangeal joints. Large joints are often affected.
Stiffness is worse after rest, e.g. on waking, and improves with
use.

Gout usually involves a single joint, such as the first metatarsophalangeal joint, but can lead to gross hand involvement
with asymmetric uric acid lumps (*tophi*) by some joints, and in
the tips of the ears.

Septic arthritis: this is important not to miss — a single, hot
painful joint.

— **Functional disability**: 'How far can you walk? Can you walk up-stairs? Is any particular movement difficult? Can you dress yourself? How long does it take? Can you work? Can you write?'

Thyroid disease

O Ask about the following points:
  — **Weight change.**
  — **Reaction to the weather**: 'Do you dislike the hot or cold weather?'
  — **Irritability**: 'Are you more or less irritable compared with a few years ago?'
  — **Diarrhoea/constipation.**
  — **Palpitations.**
  — **Dry skin or greasy hair**: 'Is your skin dry or greasy? Is your hair dry or greasy?'
  — **Depression**: 'How has your mood been?'
  — **Croaky voice.**

> *Hypothyroid* patients put on weight without increase in ap-petite, dislike cold weather, have dry skin and thin, dry hair, a puffy face, a croaky voice, are usually calm and may be depressed.
>
> *Hyperthyroid* patients may lose weight despite eating more, dislike hot weather, perspire excessively, have palpitations, a tremor, and may be agitated and tearful. Young people have predominantly nervous and heat intolerance symptoms, whereas old people tend to present with cardiac symptoms.

Past history

O **All previous illnesses or operations**, whether apparently impor-tant or not, must be included.

> For instance, a casually mentioned attack of influenza or chill may have been a manifestation of an occult infection.

O The importance of a past illness may be gained by finding out **how long the patient was in bed or off work.**

O **Complications of any previous illnesses** should be carefully enquired into and, here, leading questions are sometimes necessary.

General questions

O Ask about the following:
  - **'Have you had any serious illnesses?'**
  - **'Have you had any emotional or nervous problems?'**
  - **'Have you had any operations or admissions to hospital?'**
  - **'Have you ever**
    - **had jaundice, epilepsy, TB, hypertension, rheumatic fever or diabetes?**
    - **travelled abroad?**
    - **had allergies?'**
  - **'Have any medicines ever upset you?'**

        Allergic responses to drugs may include an itchy rash, vomiting, diarrhoea or severe illness, including jaundice. Many patients claim to be allergic but are not. An accurate description of the supposed allergic episodes is important.

  - Additional questions can be asked:
    - if the patient has high blood pressure, ask about kidney problems, if relatives have hypertension or whether he eats liquorice
    - if a possible heart attack, ask about hypertension, diabetes, diet, smoking, family history of heart disease
    - if the patient's history suggests cardiac failure, you must ask if he has had *rheumatic fever*

Patients have often had examinations for life insurance or the armed forces.

Family history

The family history gives clues to possible predisposition to illness (e.g. heart attacks) **and whether a patient may have reason to be particularly anxious about a certain disease** (e.g. mother died of cancer).

Death certificates and patient knowledge are often inaccurate. Patients may be reluctant to talk about relatives' illnesses if they were mental diseases, epilepsy or cancer.

General questions

o Ask about the following:
  - **'Are your parents alive?** Are they fit and well? What did your parents die from?'
  - **'Have you any brothers or sisters?** Are they fit and well?'
  - **'Do you have any children?** Are they fit and well?'
  - **'Is there any history of:**
    - **heart trouble?**
    - **diabetes?**
    - **high blood pressure in the family?'**

      These questions can be varied to take account of the patient's major complaint.

Personal and social history

One needs to find out what kind of person the patient is, what his home circumstances are and how his illness has affected him and his family. Your aim is to understand the patient's illness in the context of his personality and his home environment.

> Can he convalesce satisfactorily at home and at what stage? What are the consequences of his illness? Will advice, information and help be needed? An interview with a relative or friend may be very helpful.

General questions

o Ask about the following:
  - 'Are you in a relationship?': married, partnership and whether any children.
  - **Family:** 'Is everything alright at home? Do you have any family problems?'

    It may be appropriate to ask: 'Is your relationship alright? Is sex alright?' Problems may arise from physical or emotional reasons, and the patient may appreciate an opportunity to discuss worries.
  - **Accommodation:** 'Where do you live? Is it alright?'
  - **Job:** 'What is your job? Could you tell me exactly what you do? Is it satisfactory? Will your illness affect your work?'

- **Hobbies**: 'What do you do in your spare time? Do you have any social life?'
- **Alcohol**: 'How much alcohol do you drink?'

  Alcoholics usually underestimate their daily consumption. It may be helpful to go through a 'drinking day'. If there is a suspicion of a drinking problem, you can ask: 'Do you ever drink in the morning? Do you worry about controlling your drinking? Does it affect your job, home or social life?'

- **Smoking**: 'Do you smoke?' Have you ever smoked? Why did you give up? How many cigarettes, cigars or pipefuls of tobacco do you smoke a day?'

  Particularly relevant for heart or chest disease, but must always be asked.

- **Drugs**: 'Do you take any recreational drugs?'
- **Prescribed medications**: 'What pills are you taking at the moment? Have you taken any other pills in the last few months?'

  This is an extremely important question. A complete list of all drugs and doses must be obtained.

  If relevant, ask about any pets, visits abroad, previous or present exposure during working to coal dust, asbestos, etc.

The patient's ideas, concerns and expectations

Make sure that you understand the patient's main ideas, concerns and expectations. Either now, or after examining the patient, ask for example:

- **What do you think is wrong with you?**
- **What are you expecting to happen to you whilst you are in hospital?**
- **Is there something particular you would like us to do?**
- **Have you any questions?**

  The patient's main concerns may not be your main concerns. The patient may have quite different expectations of the hospital admission, or outpatient appointment, from what you assume. If you fail to address the patient's concerns he is likely to be dissatisfied, leading to difficult doctor–patient relationships and non-compliance.

Strategy

Having taken the history, you should

O **have some idea of possible diagnoses**

O **have made an assessment of the patient as a person**

O **know which systems you wish to concentrate on when examining the patient**

Further relevant questions may arise from abnormalities found on examination or investigation.

Specimen history

Mr John Smith.

Aged 52. Machine operator. Oxford.

c/o severe chest pain for 2 hours.

History of present illness

— Perfectly well until 6 months ago.

— Began to notice central, dull chest ache, occasionally felt in the jaw, coming on when walking about 1 km (1/2 mile), worse when going uphill and worse in cold weather. When he stopped, the pain went off after 2 minutes.

— Glyceryl trinitrate spray relieved the pain rapidly.

— Last month the pain came on with less exercise after 100 yards.

— Today at 10 a.m. whilst sitting at work the chest pain came on without provocation. It was the worst pain he had ever experienced in his life and he thought he was going to die.

— The pain was central, crushing in nature, radiating to the left arm and neck and with it a feeling of nausea and sweating. The patient was rushed to hospital where he received an intravenous injection of diamorphine, which rapidly relieved the pain, and intravenous streptokinase. An electrocardiogram confirmed a myocardial infarction and the patient was admitted to the coronary care unit.

— The patient had noticed very mild breathlessness on exertion for 3 months, but had not experienced palpitations, dizziness, breathlessness on lying flat, ankle swelling or coughing. On one occasion, however, 2 weeks ago the patient had woken with a suffocating feeling and had had to sit on the edge of the bed and subsequently open the bedroom window in order to get his breath. This had not recurred and he did not report it to his doctor.

Functional enquiry

Respiratory system (RS):
- morning cough over the last 3—4 winters with production of a small amount of clear sputum
- no haemoptysis

Gastrointestinal (GI):
- occasional mild indigestion
- bowels regular
- appetite normal
- no other abnormalities

Genitourinary (GU):
- no difficulties with micturition
- normal sex life

Nervous system (NS):
- infrequent frontal headaches at the end of a hectic day
- otherwise no abnormalities
- no psychiatric symptoms

Past medical history

Fifteen years ago, appendicectomy. No complications.
No other operations or serious illnesses.
No history of rheumatic fever, nephritis or hypertension.
Never been abroad.

Family history

Father died aged 73 — 'heart attack'.
Mother died aged 71 — 'cancer'.
Two brothers fit and well (aged 48 and 46).
Two sons (aged 23, 25), both fit and well.
No family history of diabetes or hypertension.

Personal and social history

Happy both at work and home. Both sons married and living in Oxford. Wife works as an office cleaner. No financial difficulties.

Smokes 20 cigarettes per day. Two pints of beer on Saturdays only.

Patient always worked as machine operator since leaving school except for 2 years in Hong Kong, where he had no illness.

Medication

Other than glyceryl trinitrate spray, no drugs currently being taken.

CHAPTER 2

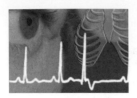

General Examination

The initial assessment of the patient will have been made whilst taking a history. The **general appearance of the patient** is the first observation, and thereafter the order of examination will vary.

The system to which the presenting symptoms refer is often examined first. Otherwise devise your own routine, examining each part of the body in turn, covering all systems. An example is:

- **general appearance**
- **alertness, mood, general behaviour**
- **hands and nails**
- **radial pulse**
- **axillary nodes**
- **cervical lymph nodes**
- **facies, eyes, tongue**
- **jugular venous pressure**
- **heart, breasts**
- **respiratory system**
- **spine (whilst patient is sitting forward)**
- **abdomen, including femoral pulses**
- **legs**
- **nervous system including fundi**
- **rectal or pelvic examination**
- **gait**

Whichever part of the body one is examining, one should always use the same routine:

1 **Inspection.**
2 **Palpation.**

3 **Percussion.**
4 **Auscultation.**

General inspection

The beginning of the examination is a careful observation of the patient as a whole. Note the following:

O **Does the patient look ill?**
- what age does he look?
- febrile, dehydrated
- alert, confused, drowsy
- cooperative, happy, sad, resentful
- fat, muscular, wasted
- in pain or distressed

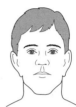

Hands

Note the following:

O **Temperature:**
- unduly cold hands —? *low cardiac output*
- unduly warm hands —? *high-output state*, e.g. *thyrotoxicosis*
- cold and sweaty —? anxiety or other causes of *sympathetic overreactivity*, e.g. *hypoglycaemia*

O **Peripheral cyanosis.**
O **Raynaud's.**
O **Nicotine staining.**

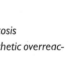

Normal

O **Nails:**
- bitten
- leukonychia—white nails
  —can occur in *cirrhosis*
- koilonychia—misshapen, concave nails (Plate 2d)
  —can occur in *iron-deficiency anaemia*
- clubbing—loss of angle at base of nail (Plate 2a)

Koilonychia

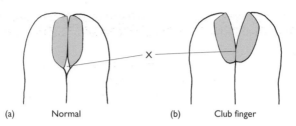

(a)   Normal   (b)   Club finger

(a) Fingers held together — space seen at X as a result of normal angles in the fingers. (b) Positive Schamroth's sign — space is lost as a result of clubbing.

Nail clubbing occurs in specific diseases:

> Heart: *infectious endocarditis, cyanotic congenital heart disease.*
> Lungs: *carcinoma of the bronchus* (*chronic infection: abscess; bronchiectasis, e.g. cystic fibrosis; empyema); fibrosing alveolitis* (not chronic bronchitis).
> Liver: *cirrhosis.*
> *Crohn's disease.*
> *Congenital.*

Clubbing

— splinter haemorrhages — occur in *infectious endocarditis* but are more common in people doing manual work
— pitting — *psoriasis*
— onycholysis — separation of nail from nail bed *psoriasis, thyrotoxicosis*
— paronychia — pustule in lateral nail fold

Splinter haemorrhages

o **Palms:**
  — erythema — can be normal, also occurs with *chronic liver disease, pregnancy*
  — Dupuytren's contracture (Plate 4c) — tethering of skin in palm to flexor tendon of fourth finger

o **Joints:**
  — symmetrical swellings occur in *rheumatoid arthritis* (Plate 2e)
  — asymmetrical swellings occur in *gout* (Plate 2f) and *osteoarthritis*

Skin

Inspection of skin

- distribution of any lesions from end of bed
- examine close up with palpation of skin
- remember mucous membranes, hair and nails

O **Colour:**
- pigmented apart from racial pigmentation or suntan — examine buccal mucosa
- if appears jaundiced — examine sclerae
- if pale — examine conjunctivae for anaemia

O **Skin texture:**
- ? normal for age — becomes thinner from age 50
- thin, e.g. *Cushing's syndrome, hypothyroid, hypopituitary, malnutrition, liver or renal failure*
- thick, e.g. *acromegaly, androgen excess*
- dry, e.g. *hypothyroid*
- tethered, e.g. *scleroderma* of fingers, attached to underlying breast tumour

O **Rash:**
- what is it like? Describe precisely

Inspection of lesions

- distribution of lesions:
    - symmetrical or asymmetrical
    - peripheral or mainly on trunk
    - maximal on light-exposed sites
    - pattern of contact with known agents, e.g. shoes, gloves, cosmetics
- number and size of lesions
- look at an early lesion
- discrete or confluent
- pattern of lesions, e.g. linear, annular, serpiginous (like a snake), reticular (like a net)
- is edge well-demarcated?

- colour
- surface, e.g. scaly, shiny

Palpation of lesions

- flat, impalpable — *macular* (Plate 3c)
- raised
    papular: in skin, localized
    plaque: larger, e.g. >0.5 cm
    nodules: deeper in dermis, persisting more than 3 days
    wheal: oedema fluid, transient, less than 3 days
    vesicles: contain fluid (Plate 3e)
    bullae: large vesicles, e.g. >0.5 cm
    pustular
- deep in dermis — *nodules*
- temperature
- tender?
- blanches on pressure — most erythematous lesions, e.g. *drug rash*, *telangiectasia*, dilated capillaries
- does not blanch on pressure
        Purpura or *petechiae* are small discrete microhaemorrhages approximately 1 mm across, red, non-tender macules.
        If palpable, suggests *vasculitis* (Plate 3d).
        Senile purpura local haemorrhages are from minor traumas in thin skin of hands or forearms. Flat purple/brown lesions.
- hard
    - sclerosis, e.g. *scleroderma* of fingers (Plate 4b)
    - infiltration, e.g. *lymphoma* or *cancer*
    - scars

Enquire about the time course of any lesion

- 'How long has it been there?'
    - 'Is it fixed in size and position? Does it come and go?'
    - 'Is it itchy, sore, tender or anaesthetic?'
Knowledge of the differential diagnosis will indicate other questions:
    dermatitis of hand — contact with chemicals or plants, wear and tear;

ulcer of toe — *arterial disease*, *diabetes mellitus*, *neuropathy*;
pigmentation and ulcer of lower medial leg — *varicose veins*.

Common diseases

Acne	Pilar-sebaceous follicular inflammation — papules and pustules on face and upper trunk, blackheads (*comedones*), cysts.
Basal cell carcinoma (rodent ulcer) (Plate 5e)	Shiny papule with rolled border and capillaries on surface. Can have a depressed centre or ulcerate.
Bullae	Blisters due to burns, infection of the skin, allergy or, rarely, autoimmune diseases affecting adhesion within epidermis (*pemphigus*) or at the epidermal–dermal junction (*pemphigoid*).
Café-au-lait patches	Permanent discrete brown macules of varying size and shape. If large and numerous, suggests neurofibromatosis.
Drug eruptions (Plate 3c)	Usually macular, symmetrical distribution. Can be urticaria, eczematous and various forms, including erythema multiforme or erythema nodosum (see below).
Eczema (Plate 3b)	*Atopic dermatitis:* dry skin, red, plaques, commonly on the face, antecubital and popliteal fossae, with fine scales, vesicles and scratch marks secondary to *pruritus* (itching). Often associated with *asthma* and *hayfever*. Family history of atopy. *Contact dermatitis:* may be irritant or allergic. Red, scaly plaques with vesicles in acute stages.
Erythema multiforme	Symmetrical, widespread inflammatory 0.5–1 cm macules/papules, often with central blister. Can be confluent. Usually on hands and feet: *drug reactions*

	viral infections
	no apparent cause
	Stevens–Johnson syndrome — with mucosal desquamation involving genitalia, mouth and conjunctivae, with fever.
Erythema nodosum (Plate 3f)	Tender, localized, red, diffusely raised, 2–4 cm nodules in anterior shins. Due to: *streptococcal infection*, e.g. with *rheumatic fever* *primary tuberculosis* and other infections *sarcoid* *inflammatory bowel disease* *drug reactions* *no apparent cause*
Fungus	Red, annular, scaly area of skin. When involving the nails, they become thickened with loss of compact structure.
Herpes infection (Plate 6f)	Clusters of vesicopustules which crust, recurs at the same site, e.g. lips, buttocks.
Impetigo	Spreading pustules and yellow crusts from staphylococcal infection.
Malignant melanoma	Usually irregular pigmented, papule or plaque, superficial or thick with irregular edge, enlarging with tendency to bleed.
Psoriasis (Plate 3a)	Symmetrical eruption: chronic, discrete, red plaques with silvery scales. Gentle scraping easily induces bleeding. Often affects scalp, elbows and knees. Nails may be pitted. Familial and precipitated by streptococcal sore throats or skin trauma.
Scabies	Mite infection: itching with 2–4 mm tunnels in epidermis, e.g. in webs of fingers, wrists, genitalia.
Squamous cell carcinoma	Warty localized thickening, may ulcerate.
Urticaria	Transient wheal with surrounding erythema. Lasts around 24 hours. Usually allergic to

drugs, e.g. aspirin, or physical, e.g.
dermographism, cold.

Vitiligo   Permanent demarcated, depigmented white
patches due to autoimmune disease.

Mouth

O **Look at the tongue:**
— cyanosed, moist or dry

> *Cyanosis* is a reduction in the oxygenation of the blood, with
> more than 5 g/dl deoxygenated haemoglobin.
>
> **Central cyanosis** (blue tongue) denotes
> a right-to-left shunt (unsaturated blood
> appearing in systemic circulation):
> — congenital heart disease, e.g. *Fallot's
> tetralogy*
> — lung disease, e.g. *obstructive airways
> disease*

Central cyanosis

> **Peripheral cyanosis** (blue fingers,
> pink tongue) denotes inadequate
> peripheral circulation.
>   A dry tongue can mean salt
> and water deficiency (often called
> 'dehydration') but also occurs with
> mouth-breathing.

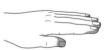
Peripheral cyanosis

O **Look at the teeth:**
— caries (exposed dentine), poor dental hygiene, false
O **Look at the gums:**
— bleeding, swollen
O **Look at: redness, exudate**
— tonsils
— pharynx: swelling, redness, ulceration
O **Smell patient's breath:**
— ketosis
— alcohol
— foetor

constipation, appendicitis

musty in liver failure

> *Ketosis* is a sweet-smelling breath occurring with *starvation* or *severe diabetes.*
>
> *Hepatic foetor* is a musty smell in *liver failure.*

Eyes

O Look at the eyes:

— *sclera*, icterus

> The most obvious demonstration of *jaundice* is the yellow sclera (Plate 1e).

— *lower lid conjunctiva*, anaemia

> *Anaemia.* If the lower lid is everted, the colour of the mucous membrane can be seen. If these are pale, the haemoglobin is usually less than 9 g/dl.

— eyelids: white/yellow deposit, *xanthelasma* (Plate 5a)

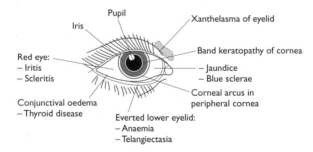

Pupil
Iris
Xanthelasma of eyelid
Band keratopathy of cornea
Red eye:
– Iritis
– Scleritis
Jaundice
– Blue sclerae
Corneal arcus in peripheral cornea
Conjunctival oedema
– Thyroid disease
Everted lower eyelid:
– Anaemia
– Telangiectasia

— puffy eyelids

> general oedema, e.g. *nephrotic syndrome*
>
> *thyroid eye disease* (Plate 1a), hyper or hypo
>
> *myxoedema* (Plate 1b)

— red eye

> *iritis*
>
> *conjunctivitis*
>
> *scleritis* or *episcleritis*
>
> *acute glaucoma*

- white line around cornea, *arcus senilis*
    common and of little significance in the elderly
    suggests *hyperlipidaemia* in younger patients (Plate 5b)
- white-band keratopathy-hypercalcaemia
    sarcoid
    parathyroid tumour or *hyperplasia*
    lung oat-cell tumour
    bone secondaries
    vitamin D excess intake
    Hypercalcaemia may give a horizontal band across exposed medial and lateral parts of cornea.

Examine the fundi

This is often done as part of the neurological system, when examining the cranial nerves. It is placed here as features cover general medicine.

O **Use ophthalmoscope**
- The patient should be sitting. Start examination at 1 m from the patient, identify red reflex and approach the patient at an angle of 15° to the patient. Approach on the same horizontal plane as patient's equator of their eye. This will bring the observer straight to the optic disc. After observing the disc examine the peripheral retina fully by following the blood vessels to and back from the four main quadrants.
    - Use your right eye for patient's right eye, left eye for patient's left eye.

O **Look at optic disc**
- normally pink rim with white 'cup' below surface of disc
- *optic atrophy*
    - disc pale: rim no longer pink
        multiple sclerosis
        after optic neuritis
        optic nerve compression, e.g. *tumour*
- papilloedema
    - disc pink, indistinct margin
    - cup disappears
    - dilated retinal veins:

increased cerebral pressure, e.g. tumour
accelerated hypertension
optic neuritis, acute stage
- glaucoma — enlarged cup, diminished rim
- new vessels — new fronds of vessels coming forward from disc;
    ischaemic diabetic retinopathy

○ **Look at arteries**
- arteries narrowed in hypertension, with increased light reflex along top of vessel
    Hypertension grading:
    1 narrow arteries
    2 'nipping' (narrowing of veins by arteries)
    3 flame-shaped haemorrhages and cotton-wool spots
    4 papilloedema.
- occlusion artery — pale retina
- occlusion vein — haemorrhages

○ **Look at retina**
- hard exudates (shiny, yellow circumscribed patches of lipid)
    diabetes
- cotton-wool spots (soft, fluffy white patches)

Hypertensive retinopathy (Plate 6a)

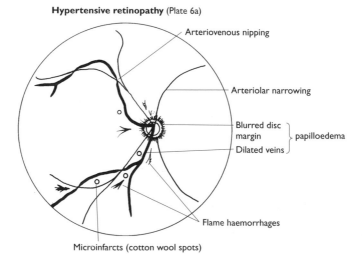

Arteriovenous nipping

Arteriolar narrowing

Blurred disc margin ⎫
                    ⎬ papilloedema
Dilated veins ⎭

Flame haemorrhages

Microinfarcts (cotton wool spots)

microinfarcts causing local swelling of nerve fibres
>   *diabetes*
>   *hypertension*
>   *vasculitis*
>   *human immunodeficiency virus* (HIV)

— small, red dots
microaneurysms — retinal capillary expansion adjacent to capillary closure
>   *diabetes*

— haemorrhages
round 'blots': haemorrhages deep in retina
larger than microaneurysms
>   *diabetes*

— flame-shaped: superficial haemorrhages along nerve fibres
>   *hypertension*
>   *gross anaemia*
>   *hyperviscosity*
>   *bleeding tendency*

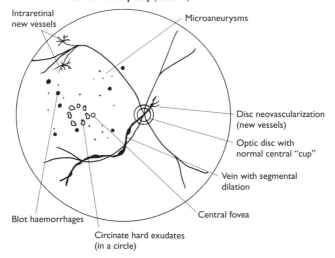

Diabetic retinopathy (Plate 6b)

Intraretinal new vessels

Microaneurysms

Disc neovascularization (new vessels)

Optic disc with normal central "cup"

Vein with segmental dilation

Blot haemorrhages

Central fovea

Circinate hard exudates (in a circle)

- Roth's spots (white-centred haemorrhages)
    - *microembolic disorder*
    - *subacute bacterial endocarditis*
- pigmentation
    - widespread
        - *retinitis pigmentosa*
    - localized
        - *choroiditis* (clumping of pigment into patches)
        - *drug toxicity*, e.g. chloroquine
    - tigroid or tabby fundus: normal variant in choroid beneath retina
- peripheral new vessels
    - *ischaemic diabetic retinopathy*
    - *retinal vein occlusion*
- medullated nerve fibres — normal variant, areas of white nerves radiating from optic disc

Examine for palpable lymph nodes

O In the neck:
- above clavicle (posterior triangle)
- medial to sternomastoid area (anterior triangle)
- submandibular (can palpate submandibular gland)
- occipital

    These glands are best felt by sitting the patient up and examining from behind. A left supraclavicular node can occur from the spread of a gastrointestinal malignancy (Virchow's node).

O In the axillae:
- abduct arm, insert your hand along lateral side of axilla, and adduct arm, thus placing your fingertips in the apex of the axilla. Palpate gently

O In the epitrochlear region:
- medial to and above elbow

O In the groins:
- over inguinal ligament

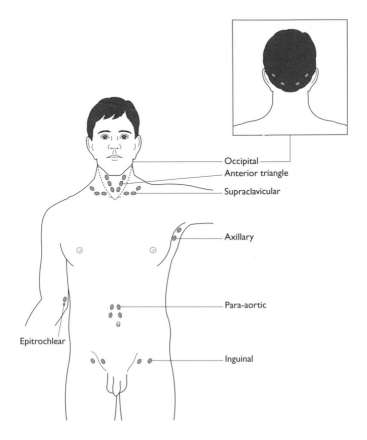

Occipital

Anterior triangle

Supraclavicular

Axillary

Para-aortic

Epitrochlear

Inguinal

○ In the abdomen:
  – usually very difficult to feel; some claim to have felt para-aortic
    nodes
        Axillae often have soft, fleshy lymph nodes.
        Groins often have small, shotty nodes.
        Generalized large, rubbery nodes suggest *lymphoma*.
        Localized hard nodes suggest *cancer*.
        Tender nodes suggest *infection*.
     If many nodes are palpable — examine spleen and look for anaemia.
     Lymphoma or *leukaemia*?

Lumps

O If there is an unusual lump, **inspect first and palpate later:**
  - **site**
  - **size** (measure in centimetres)
  - **shape**
  - **surface, edge**
  - **surroundings**
  - **fixed or mobile**
  - **consistency**, e.g. cystic or solid, soft or hard, fluctuance
  - **tender**
  - **pulsatile**
  - **auscultation**
  - **transillumination**

    A *cancer* is usually hard, non-tender, irregular, fixed to neigh-bouring tissues, and possibly ulcerating skin.

    A *cyst* may have:
  - **fluctuance**: pressure across cyst will cause it to bulge in another plane
  - **transillumination**: a light can be seen through it (usually only if room is darkened)
O Look at neighbouring lymph nodes. May find:
  - spread from cancer
  - inflamed lymph nodes from infection

Breasts

When appropriate, arrange a female chaperone, particularly when the patient is a young adult, shy or nervous.

Routine examination
O Examine the female breasts **when you examine the precordium.**
O **Inspect for asymmetry**, obvious lumps, inverted nipples, skin changes.
O **Palpate each quadrant of both breasts** with the flat of the

hand (fingers together, nearly extended with gentle pressure exerted from metacarpophalangeal joints, avoiding pressure on the nipple).

O If there are any possible lumps, proceed to a more complete examination.

Full breast examination

When patient has a symptom or a lump has been found:

O **Inspect**
  - **sitting up and ask the patient to raise hands**
  - **inspect for asymmetry** or obvious lumps
    - differing size or shape of breasts
    - nipples — symmetry
    - rashes, redness (abscess)
        Breast cancer is suggested by:
        - asymmetry
        - skin tethering
        - *peau d'orange* (oedema of skin)
        - nipple deviated or inverted

O **Palpate**
  - patient lying flat, one pillow
  - **examine each breast with flat of hand, each quadrant in turn**
  - examine bimanually if large
  - examine any lump as described on p. 39
    - is lump attached to skin or muscles?
    - examine lymph nodes (axilla and supraclavicular)
    - feel liver

Thyroid

O **Inspect**: then ask the patient to swallow, having given him a glass of water. Is there a lump? Does it move upwards on swallowing?

O **Palpate bimanually**: stand behind the patient and palpate with fingers of both hands. Is the thyroid of normal size, shape and texture?

O If a lump is felt:

— is thyroid multinodular?

— does lump feel cystic?

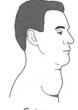

Goitre

> The thyroid is normally soft. If there is a goitre (swelling of thyroid), assess if the swelling is:
>
> — localized, e.g. *thyroid cyst, adenoma* or *carcinoma*
>
> — generalized, e.g. *autoimmune thyroiditis, thyrotoxicosis*
>
> — multinodular
>
> A swelling does not mean the gland is under- or overactive. In many cases the patient may be euthyroid. The thyroid becomes slightly enlarged in pregnancy.

- **Ask patient to swallow** — does thyroid rise normally?
- Is thyroid fixed?
- **Can you get below the lump?** If not, percuss over upper sternum for retrosternal extension
- **Are there cervical lymph nodes?**
- **If possibility of patient being thyrotoxic (Plate 1a), look for:**
  - warm hands
  - perspiration
  - tremor
  - tachycardia, sinus rhythm or atrial fibrillation
  - wide, palpable fissure or lid lag
  - thyroid bruit (on auscultation)

    > *Endocrine exophthalmos* (may be associated with thyrotoxicosis):
    >
    > — conjunctival oedema: *chemosis* (seen by gentle pressure on lower lid, pushing up a fold of conjunctiva when oedema is present)
    >
    > — proptosis: eye pushed forwards (look from above down on eyes)
    >
    > — deficient upward gaze and convergence
    >
    > — diplopia
    >
    > — papilloedema

- If possibility of patient being *hypothyroid* (Plate 1b), look for:

- dry hair and skin
- xanthelasma
- puffy face
- croaky voice
- delayed relaxation of supinator or ankle jerks

Other endocrine diseases

Acromegaly (Plate 1c)
- enlarged soft tissue of hands, feet, face
- coarse features, thick, greasy skin, large tongue (and other organs, e.g. thyroid)
- bitemporal hemianopia (from tumour pressing on optic chiasma)

Hypopituitary
- no skin pigmentation
- thin skin
- decreased secondary sexual hair or delayed puberty
- short stature (and on X-ray, delayed fusion of epiphyses)
- bitemporal hemianopia if pituitary tumour

Addison's disease
- increased skin pigmentation, including non-exposed areas, e.g. buccal pigmentation
- postural hypotension
- if female, decreased body hair

Cushing's syndrome (Plate 1d)
- truncal obesity, round, red face with hirsutism
- thin skin and bruising, pink striae, hypertension
- proximal muscle weakness

Diabetes
Diabetic complications include:
- skin lesions
    Necrobiosis lipoidica — ischaemia in skin, usually on shins,

leading to fatty replacement of dermis, covered by thin skin.

- ischaemic legs (Plate 4e)
  - diminished foot pulses
  - skin shiny blue, white or black
  - no hairs, thick nails
  - ulcers (Plate 4f)
- peripheral neuropathy
  - absent leg reflexes
  - diminished sensation
  - thick skin over unusual pressure points from dropped arch
- autonomic neuropathy
  - dry skin
- mononeuropathy
  - lateral popliteal nerve—footdrop
  - III or VI—diplopia
  - asymmetrical muscle-wasting of the upper leg
- retinopathy (Plate 6b)

Locomotor system

Normally one examines joints briefly when examining neighbouring systems. If a patient specifically complains of joint symptoms or an abnormal posture or joint is noted, a more detailed examination is needed.

General habitus

- Note the following:
  - is the patient unduly tall or short? Measure height and span
  - are all limbs, spine and skull of normal size and shape?
    - normal person:
      height = span
      crown to pubis = pubis to heel
    - long limbs:
      Marfan's syndrome
      eunuchoid during growth

— *collapsed vertebrae:*
    span > height
    pubis to heel > crown to pubis
— is the posture normal?
— curvature of the spine:
    flexion: *kyphosis*
    extension: *lordosis*
    lateral: *scoliosis*
— is the gait normal?

Flexion

Extension

Lateral

Observing the patient walking is a vital part of examination of the locomotor system and neurological system.

Painful gait, transferring weight quickly off a painful limb, bobbing up and down—an abnormal rhythm of gait.

Painless abnormal gait may be from:
    short leg (bobs up and down with equal-length steps)
    stiff joint (lifts pelvis to prevent foot dragging on ground)
    weak ankle (high stepping gait to avoid toes catching on ground)
    weak knee (locks knee straight before putting foot on the ground)
    weak hip (sways sideways using trunk muscles to lift pelvis and to swing leg through)
    uncoordinated gait (arms are swung as counterbalances)
    hysterical or malingering causes

Look for abnormal wear on shoes.

Inspection
O Inspect the joints before you touch them.
O Look at:
— skin
    redness—inflammation
    scars—old injury
    bruising—recent injury
— soft tissues
    muscle wasting—old injury

swelling—injury/inflammation
- bones
    deformity—compare with other side
        Varus: bent in to midline
        Valgus: bent out from midline

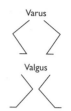
Varus

Valgus

O Assess whether an isolated joint is affected, or if there is polyarthritis.

O If there is polyarthritis, note if it is symmetrical or asymmetrical.

O Compare any abnormal findings with the other side.

Arthritis—swollen, hot, tender, painful joint.

Arthropathy—swollen but not hot and tender.

Arthralgia—painful, e.g. on movement, without being swollen.

Swelling may also be due to an effusion, thickening of the periarticular tissues, enlargement of the ends of bones (e.g. *pulmonary osteopathy*) or complete disorganization of the joint without pain (*Charcot's joint*).

Palpation

O Before you touch any joint ask the patient to tell you if it is painful.

O Feel for:
- warmth
- tenderness
    - watch patient's face for signs of discomfort
    - locate signs of tenderness—soft tissue or bone
- swelling or displacement
- fluctuation (effusion)

An inflamed joint is usually generally tender. Localized tenderness may be mechanical in origin, e.g. ligament tear. Joint effusion may occur with an arthritis or local injury.

Movement

Test the range of movement of the joint both actively and passively. This must be done **gently**.

O **Active**—how far can the patient move the joint through its range?

Do not seize limb and move it until patient complains.

O **Passive**—if range is limited, can you further increase the range of movement?

> Abduction: movement from central axis.
> Adduction: movement to central axis.

— Is the passive range of movement similar to the active range?

> Limitation of the range of movement of a joint may be due to pain, muscle spasms, contracture, inflammation or thickening of the capsules or periarticular structures, effusions into the joint space, bony or cartilaginous outgrowths or painful conditions not connected with the joint.

O **Resisted movement**—ask patient to bend joint while you resist movement. How much force can be developed?

O **Hold your hand round the joint** whilst it is moving. A grating or creaking sensation (*crepitus*) may be felt.

> Crepitus is usually associated with *osteoarthritis*.

Summary of signs of common illnesses

Osteoarthritis
— 'wear and tear' of a specific joint—usually large joints
— common in elderly or after trauma to joint
— often involves joints of the lower limbs and is asymmetrical
— often in the lumbar or cervical spine
— aches after use, with deep, boring pain at night
— Heberden's nodes—osteophytes on terminal interphalangeal joints

Rheumatoid arthritis (Plate 2e)
Characteristically:
— a polyarthritis
— symmetrical, inflamed if active
— involves proximal interphalangeal and metacarpophalangeal joints of hands with ulnar deviation of fingers
— involves any large joint
— muscle wasting from disuse atrophy
— rheumatoid nodules on extensor surface of elbows
— may include other signs, e.g. with splenomegaly it is *Felty's syndrome*

Gout (Plate 2f)

Characteristically:

- asymmetrical
- inflamed first metatarsophalangeal joint (big toe) —*podagra*
- involves any joint in hand, often with tophus — hard round lump of urate by joint
- tophi on ears

Psoriasis (Plate 3a)

- particularly involves terminal interphalangeal joints, hips and knees
- often with pitted nails of psoriasis as well as skin lesions

Ankylosing spondylitis

- painful, stiff spine
- later fixed in flexed position
- hips and other joints can be involved

System-oriented examination

On a ward round in outpatients, or 'short cases' in examinations, it is common to be asked to examine a single system. It is important to have set examination schedules in your mind, so you do not miss any salient features. You may choose a different order from those suggested if it helps you. Learn the major features by rote.

At the end of each examination chapter is such a list.

'Examine the face'

- observe skin: *rodent ulcer*
- upper face: *Paget's disease, balding, myopathy, Bell's palsy*
- eyes: *anaemia, jaundice, thyrotoxicosis, myxoedema, xanthelasma, ptosis, eye palsies, Horner's syndrome*
- lower face: *steroid therapy, acromegaly, Parkinson's disease, hemiparesis, parotid tumour, thyroid enlargement*

'Examine the eyes'

- observe: *jaundice, anaemia, arcus, ptosis, Horner's syndrome*
- examine:
  - check if patient is blind — beware of glass eye
  - movements of the eyes
    - amblyopia or palsy
    - diplopia, nystagmus/false image
  - visual acuity
  - visual fields
  - pupils: light and accommodation reflexes
  - fundi: disc, arteries and veins, retina, particularly fovea

'Examine the neck'

- inspect from front and side
  - thyroid (ask patient to swallow)
  - lymph nodes
  - raised jugular venous pressure
  - lymph glands
  - other swellings
- inspect from front
  - examine neck veins
  - feel carotid arteries
  - auscultate bruits over thyroid and carotid arteries
  - check trachea is central

CHAPTER 3

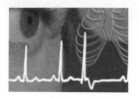

Examination of the Cardiovascular System

General examination

o **Examine:**
- clubbing of fingernails

   Clubbing in relation to the heart suggests *infective endocarditis* or *cyanotic heart disease* (Plate 2b).
- cold hands with blue nails — poor perfusion, peripheral cyanosis
- tongue for central cyanosis
- conjunctivae for anaemia
- signs of dyspnoea or distress

   Assess the degree of breathlessness by checking if *dyspnoea* occurs on undressing, talking, at rest or when lying flat (*orthopnoea*).
- xanthomata:

   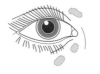

   - *xanthelasma* (common) — intracutaneous yellow cholesterol deposits occur around the eyes — normal or with *hyper-lipidaemia* (Plate 5a)
   - *xanthoma* (uncommon):

      hypercholesterolaemia — tendon deposits (hands and Achilles tendon) or tuberous xanthomata at elbows (Plate 5c)

      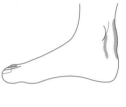

      hypertriglyceridaemia — eruptive xanthoma, small yellow deposits on buttocks and extensor surfaces, each with a red halo

Palpate the radial pulse

Feel the radial pulse just medial to the radius, with two forefingers.

○ **Pulse rate.**

Take over 15 seconds (smart Alecs count for 6 seconds and multiply by 10):
- — *tachycardia* >100 beats/min
- — *bradycardia* <50 beats/min

○ **Rhythm:**
- — regular

   Normal variation on breathing: *sinus arrhythmia*

- — regularly irregular

   pulsus bigeminus, coupled extra-systoles (digoxin toxicity)
   Wenckebach heart block

- — irregularly irregular

   multiple extrasystoles
   atrial fibrillation

   Check apical rate by auscultation for true heart rate, as small pulses are not transmitted to radial pulse.

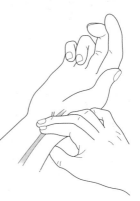

○ **Waveform of the pulse:**
- — normal (1)
- — slow rising and plateau—moderate or severe *aortic stenosis* (2)
- — collapsing pulse—pulse pressure greater than diastolic pressure, e.g. *aortic incompetence*, elderly *arteriosclerotic* patient or *gross anaemia* (3)
- — bisferiens—moderate *aortic stenosis* with severe *incompetence* (4)
- — pulsus paradoxus—pulse weaker or disappears on inspiration, e.g. *constrictive pericarditis, tamponade, status asthmaticus* (5)

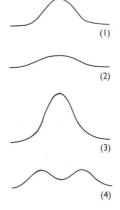

(1)

(2)

(3)

(4)

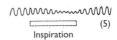

(5)

Inspiration

○ **Volume:**
  — small volume—low cardiac output
  — large volume
        carbon dioxide retention
        thyrotoxicosis
○ **Stiffness of the vessel wall:**
  — in the elderly, a stiff, strongly pulsating, palpable 5–6 cm radial artery indicates *arteriosclerosis*, a hardening of the walls of the artery that is common with aging
        is not atheroma
        is associated with systolic hypertension
○ **Pulsus alternans.**
        A difference of 20 mmHg systolic blood pressure between consecutive beats signifies poor left ventricular function. This needs to be measured with a sphygmomanometer.

Take the blood pressure

  — Wrap the cuff neatly and tightly around either upper arm. The patient should be seated with the arm at the level of the heart.
  — Gently inflate the cuff until the radial artery is no longer palpable.
  — Using the stethoscope, listen over the brachial artery for the pulse to appear as you drop the pressure slowly (3–4 mm/s).
○ Systolic blood pressure: **appearance of sounds**
        — **Korotkoff phase 1**
○ Diastolic blood pressure: **disappearance of sounds**
        — **Korotkoff phase 5**
Use large cuff for fat arms (circumference >30 cm) so that inflatable cuff >1/2 arm circumference.

Beware auscultatory gap with sounds disappearing mid-systole. If sounds go to zero, use Korotkoff phase 4.

        In adults, ~>140/85 is the current guideline in non-diabetic and ~>130/80 in diabetic patients. The patient may be nervous when first examined and the blood pressure may be falsely high. Take it again at the end of the examination.

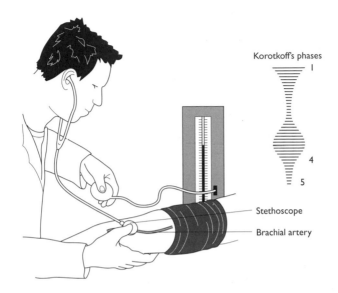

Korotkoff's phases

Stethoscope

Brachial artery

Wide pulse pressure (e.g. 160/30 mmHg) suggests *aortic incompetence.*

Narrow pulse pressure (e.g. 95/80 mmHg) suggests *aortic stenosis.*

Difference of >20 mmHg systolic between arms suggests *arterial occlusion,* e.g. *dissecting aneurysm* or *atheroma.*

Difference of 10 mmHg is found in 25% of healthy subjects.

The variable pulse from atrial fibrillation means a precise blood pressure cannot easily be obtained.

Jugular venous pressure

o Observe the height of the jugular venous pressure (JVP).

Lie the patient down, resting at approximately 45° to the horizontal with his head on pillows, and shine a torch at an angle across the neck.

○ **Look at the veins in the neck.**
  — internal jugular vein not directly visible: pulse diffuse, medial or deep to sternomastoid
  — external jugular vein: pulse lateral to sternomastoid. Only informative if pulsating
○ **Assess vertical height** in centimetres above the manubriosternal angle, using the pulsating external jugular vein or upper limit of internal jugular pulsation.

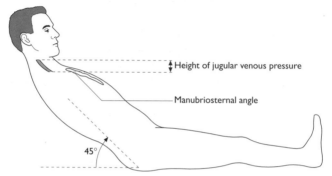

Height of jugular venous pressure

Manubriosternal angle

45°

The **external jugular vein** is often more readily visible but may be obstructed by its tortuous course, and is less reliable than the internal jugular pulse.

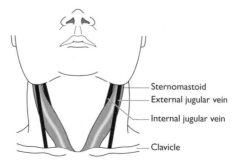

Sternomastoid
External jugular vein
Internal jugular vein

Clavicle

The **internal jugular vein** is sometimes very difficult to see. Its pulsation may be confused with the cartoid artery but it:

- has a complex pulsation
- moves on respiration and decreases on inspiration except in tamponade
- cannot be palpated
- can be obliterated by pressure on base of neck

> The **hepatojugular reflux** is checked by firm pressure with the flat of the right hand over the liver, while watching the JVP.
>
> Compression on the dilated hepatic veins increases the JVP by 2 cm.
>
> If the JVP is found to be raised above the manubriosternal angle and pulsating, it implies *right heart failure*. Look for the other signs, i.e. pitting oedema and large tender liver. Sometimes the JVP is so raised it can be missed, except that the ears waggle.
>
> Dilated neck veins with no pulsation suggest *non-cardiac obstruction* (e.g. carcinoma bronchus causing superior caval obstruction or a kinked external jugular vein).
>
> If the venous pressure rises on inspiration (it normally falls), *constrictive pericarditis* or *pericardial effusion* causing *tamponade* must be considered.

O **Observe the character of JVP.** Try to ascertain the waveform of the JVP. It should be a double pulsation consisting of:

- a-wave atrial contraction—ends synchronous with carotid artery pulse c
- v-wave atrial filling—when the tricuspid valve is closed by ventricular contraction —with and just after carotid pulse

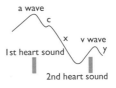

> Large a waves are caused by obstruction to flow from the right atrium due to stiffness of the right ventricle from hypertrophy:
> *pulmonary hypertension*
> *pulmonary stenosis*
> *tricuspid stenosis*
> Absent a wave in *atrial fibrillation*.

Large v waves are caused by regurgitation of blood through an *incompetent tricuspid valve* during ventricular contraction.

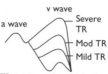

TR = tricuspid regurgitation

A sharp y descent occurs in *constrictive pericarditis*.

Cannon waves (giant a waves) occur in *complete heart block* when the right atrium occasionally contracts against a closed tricuspid valve.

The precordium

O **Inspect the precordium for abnormal pulsation.**

A large left ventricle may easily be seen on the left side of the chest, sometimes in the axilla.

O **Palpate the apex beat.**

— Feel for the point furthest out and down where the pulsation can still be distinctly felt.

O **Measure the position.**

— Which space, counting down from the second space which lies below the second rib (opposite the manubriosternal angle).

— Laterally in centimetres from the midline.

— Describe the apex beat in relation to the mid clavicular line, anterior axillary line and mid axillary line.

The normal position of the apex beat is in the fifth left intercostal space on the mid clavicular line.

O **Assess character.**

Try to judge if an enlarged heart is

— **feeble** (dilated) or

— **stronger** than usual (left or right ventricle hypertrophy or both)

Thrusting displaced apex beat occurs with volume overload: an active, large stroke volume ventricle, e.g. *mitral* or *aortic incompetence*, *left-to-right shunt* or *cardiomyopathy*.

Sustained apex beat occurs with pressure overload in

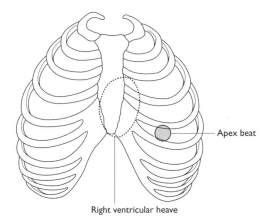

Apex beat

Right ventricular heave

aortic stenosis and *gross hypertension*. Stroke volume is normal or reduced.

Tapping apex beat (palpable first heart sound) occurs in *mitral stenosis*.

Diffuse pulsation asynchronous with apex beat occurs with a *left ventricular aneurysm* — a dyskinetic apex beat.

Impalpable — obesity, overinflated chest due to COPD, pericardial effusion.

○ **Palpate firmly the left border of the sternum.**
  — Use the flat of your hand.
    A heave suggests *right ventricular hypertrophy*.
○ **Palpate all over the precordium with the flat of hand for thrills (palpable murmurs).**

N.B. If by now you have found an abnormality in the cardiovascular system, think of possible causes before you listen.
For example, if left ventricle is forceful:
  — ?Hypertension — was blood pressure (BP) raised?
  — ?Aortic stenosis or incompetence — was pulse character normal? Will there be a murmur?
  — ?Mitral incompetence — will there be a murmur?
  — ?Thyrotoxicosis or anaemia.

Auscultation

○ **Listen over the four main areas of the heart** and in each area concentrate in order on:
  - **heart sounds**
  - **added sounds**
  - **murmurs**

Keep to this order when listening or describing what you have heard, or you will miss or forget important findings.

The four main areas are:
- **apex, mitral area** (and axilla if there is a murmur)
- **tricuspid area**
- **aortic area** (and neck if there is a murmur)
- **pulmonary area**

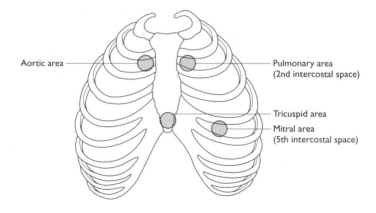

Aortic area ——

Pulmonary area
(2nd intercostal space)

Tricuspid area

Mitral area
(5th intercostal space)

These areas represent where one hears heart sounds and murmurs associated with these valves. They do not represent the surface markings of the valves.

If you hear little, turn the patient half left, and listen over apex (having palpated for it).

The diaphragm filters out low-frequency sounds, so the bell should be used for mitral stenosis.

You may find it helpful to try to imitate what you think you hear!

Normal heart sounds

I Sudden cessation of mitral and tricuspid flow due to valve closure

- loud in *mitral stenosis*
- soft in *mitral incompetence, aortic stenosis, left bundle-branch block*
- variable in *complete heart block* and *atrial fibrillation*

II Sudden cessation of aortic and pulmonary flow due to valve closure — usually split (see below)

- loud in *hypertension*
- soft in *aortic* or *pulmonary stenosis*
- wide normal split — *right bundle-branch block*
- wide fixed split — *atrial septal defect*

Added sounds

III Rapid ventricular filling sound in early diastole.

> Often **normal** until about 30 years, then probably means *heart failure, fibrosed ventricle* or *constrictive pericarditis*.

IV Atrial contraction inducing ventricular filling towards the end of the diastole.

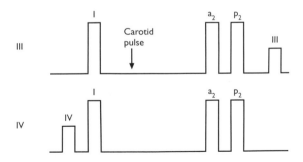

> May be normal under age 20 and in athletes, but suggests increased atrial load. Not as serious a prognosis as a third heart sound.

Canter rhythm (often termed **gallop**) with tachycardia gives the following cadences:

III: Tum——te—tum   or   **K**en——**tucky** (k = first heart sound)
IV: te–Tum——te   or   **T**enne——**ss**ee (n = first heart sound)

Opening snap

- Mitral valve normally opens silently after second heart sound.
- In *mitral stenosis*, sudden movement of rigid valve makes a click, after second heart sound (Fig. 3.1).

Ejection click

- Aortic valve normally opens silently.
- In *aortic stenosis or sclerosis*, can open with a click after first heart sound.

Splitting of second heart sound

Ask patients to take deep breaths in and out. Blood is drawn into the thorax during inspiration and then on to the right ventricle. There is temporarily more blood in the right ventricle than the left ventricle, and the right ventricle takes fractionally longer to empty.

Splitting is best heard during first two or three beats of inspiration. **Do not** ask patient to **hold** breath in or out when assessing splitting.

Paradoxical splitting occurs in *aortic stenosis* and *left bundle-branch block*.

In both these conditions (Fig. 3.2) the left ventricle takes longer to empty, thus delaying a_2 until after p_2. During inspiration p_2 occurs later and the sounds draw closer together.

Murmurs

Use the diaphragm of the stethoscope for most high-pitched sounds or murmurs (e.g. aortic incompetence) and the bell for low-pitched murmurs (e.g. mitral stenosis). Note the following:

O **Timing systolic or diastolic** (compare with finger on carotid pulse) (Fig. 3.1).
O **Site and radiation**, e.g.:
   - mitral incompetence → axilla
   - aortic stenosis → carotids and apex
   - aortic incompetence → sternum

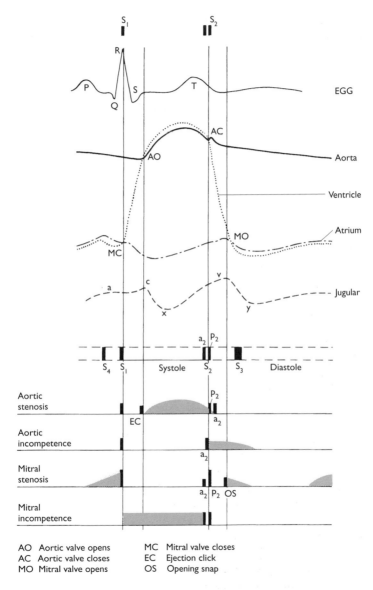

AO   Aortic valve opens   MC   Mitral valve closes
AC   Aortic valve closes   EC   Ejection click
MO   Mitral valve opens   OS   Opening snap

Fig. 3.1 Relation of murmurs to pressure changes and valve movements.

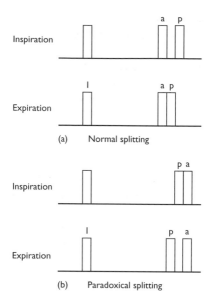

Fig. 3.2 (a) Normal and (b) paradoxical splitting.

○ **Character**
 − loud or soft
 − pitch, e.g. squeaking or rumbling, 'scratchy' = pericardial or pleural
 − length
   − pansystolic, throughout systole
   − early diastolic, e.g. aortic or pulmonary incompetence
   − mid systolic, e.g. aortic stenosis or flow murmur
   − mid diastolic, e.g. mitral stenosis
○ **Relation to posture**
 − sit forward — aortic incompetence louder
 − lie left side — mitral stenosis louder
○ **Relation to respiration**
 − inspiration increases the murmur of a right heart lesion
 − expiration increases the murmur of a left heart lesion
 − variable — pericardial rub

○ **Relation to exercise**
   — increases the murmur of mitral stenosis

Optimal position for hearing murmurs (Fig. 3.3)

○ **Mitral stenosis** — the patient lies on left side, arm above head; listen with bell at apex. Murmur is louder after exercise, e.g. repeated touching of toes from lying position that increases cardiac output.

○ **Aortic incompetence** — the patient sits forward after deep inspiration; listen with diaphragm at lower left sternal edge.

N.B. Murmurs alone do not make the diagnosis. Take other signs into consideration, e.g. arterial or venous pulses, blood pressure, apex or heart sounds.

Loudness is often not proportional to severity of disease, and in some situations length of murmur is more important, e.g. mitral stenosis.

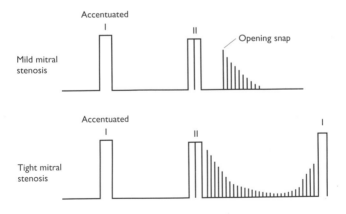

○ For completion:
   — **auscultate base of lungs** for crepitations from left ventricular failure
   — **peripheral pulses** (palpate and listen for bruits)
   — **palpate liver** — smooth, tender, enlarged in right heart failure
   — **peripheral oedema** — ankle/sacral

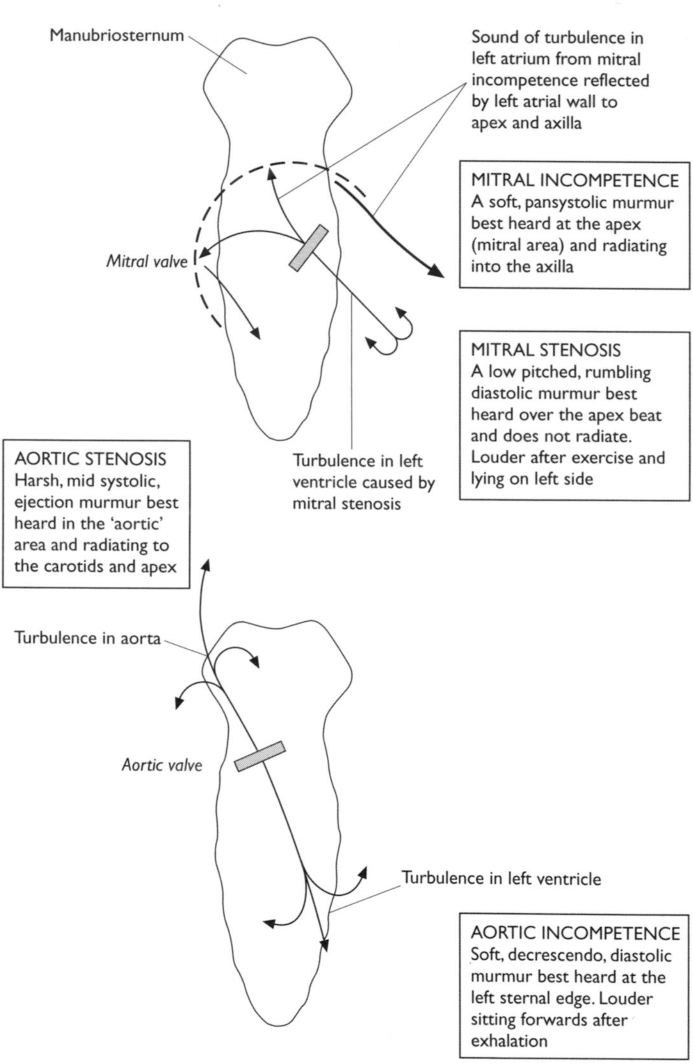

Manubriosternum

Sound of turbulence in left atrium from mitral incompetence reflected by left atrial wall to apex and axilla

MITRAL INCOMPETENCE
A soft, pansystolic murmur best heard at the apex (mitral area) and radiating into the axilla

Mitral valve

MITRAL STENOSIS
A low pitched, rumbling diastolic murmur best heard over the apex beat and does not radiate. Louder after exercise and lying on left side

AORTIC STENOSIS
Harsh, mid systolic, ejection murmur best heard in the 'aortic' area and radiating to the carotids and apex

Turbulence in left ventricle caused by mitral stenosis

Turbulence in aorta

Aortic valve

Turbulence in left ventricle

AORTIC INCOMPETENCE
Soft, decrescendo, diastolic murmur best heard at the left sternal edge. Louder sitting forwards after exhalation

Fig. 3.3 Radiation of sound from turbulent blood flow.

Summary of timing of murmurs

Ejection systolic murmur
aortic stenosis or *sclerosis* (same murmur, due to stiffness of valve cusps and aortic walls, with normal pulse pressure)
   aortic sclerosis is present in 50% of 50-year-olds
pulmonary stenosis
atrial septal defect
Fallot's syndrome — right outflow tract obstruction

Pansystolic murmur
mitral regurgitation
tricuspid regurgitation
ventricular septal defect

Late systolic murmur
mitral valve prolapse (click–murmur syndrome)
hypertrophic cardiomyopathy
coarction aorta (extending in diastole to a 'machinery murmur')

Early diastolic murmur
aortic regurgitation
pulmonary regurgitation
Graham Steell murmur in *pulmonary hypertension* (see p. 70)

Mid–late diastolic murmur
mitral stenosis
tricuspid stenosis
Austin Flint murmur in *aortic incompetence* (see p. 69)
left atrial myxoma (variable — can also give other murmurs)

Signs of left and right ventricular failure
Left heart failure
— Dyspnoea.
— Basal crepitations.

   — Fourth heart sound, or third in older patients.

O Sit the patient forward and listen at the bases of the lungs with the diaphragm of the stethoscope for fine crepitations.

> Fine crepitations are caused by alveoli opening on inspiration. When a patient has been recumbent for a while, alveoli tend to collapse in the normal lung. On taking a deep breath crepitations will be heard but do not mean pulmonary oedema. Ask the patient to cough. If crepitations continue after this, pulmonary oedema may be present.

Right heart failure

   — Raised JVP.

   — Enlarged tender liver (see later).

   — Pitting oedema.

O With the patient sitting forward, look for swelling over the sacral area. If there is, push your thumb into the swelling and see if you leave an indentation. If you do, this is called pitting oedema.

O Check both ankles for pitting oedema.

> Oedema (fluid) collects at the most dependent part of the body. A patient who is mostly sitting will have ankle oedema while a patient who is lying will have predominantly sacral oedema.

Functional result

O Having ascertained the basic pathology (e.g. *myocardial infarction*, *aortic stenosis*, *pericarditis*), make an assessment of the functional result.

   — **History.** How far can the patient walk, etc.

   — **Examination.** Evidence of:

      — cardiac enlargement (hypertrophy or dilatation)

      — heart failure

      — arrhythmias

      — pulmonary hypertension

      — cyanosis

      — endocarditis

   — **Investigations.** For example:

- chest X-ray
- electrocardiogram (ECG)
- treadmill exercise test with ECG for ischaemia
- echocardiograph — sonar 'radar' of heart, for muscle and ventricle size, muscle contractility and ejection fraction, valve function
- 24-hour ECG tape for arrhythmias
- cardiac catheterization for pressure measurements, blood oxygenation and angiogram
- radioactive scan — to image live, ischaemic or dead cardiac muscle

Summary of common illnesses

Mitral stenosis
- small pulse — fibrillating?
- JVP only raised if heart failure
- RV_{++} LVo tapping apex
- loud I. Loud p_2 if pulmonary hypertension
- opening snap (os)
- mid diastolic murmur at apex only (low-pitched rumbling)
  - severity indicated by early opening snap and long murmur
  - best heard with the patient in left lateral position, in expiration with the stethoscope bell, particularly after exercise has increased cardiac output
  - presystolic accentuation of murmur (absent if atrial fibrillation and stiff cusps)
- sounds 'ta ta rooofoo T'
  from II os murmur I

Mitral incompetence
- fibrillating?
- JVP only raised if heart failure
- RV_+ LV_{++} systolic thrill
- soft I. Loud p_2 if pulmonary hypertension
- pansystolic murmur apex $\rightarrow$ axilla

Mitral valve prolapse

— mid systolic click, late systolic murmur

— posterior cusp—murmur apex → axilla

— anterior cusp—murmur apex → aortic area

There are three stages:

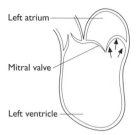

Left atrium

Mitral valve

Left ventricle

Click from billowing of cusp – larger than other cusp – may occur in 10% of females

Heard best on standing

mid-systolic click

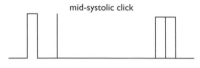

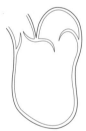

Click/late systolic murmur. After 'click', prolapsing cusp allows regurgitation

mid-systolic click

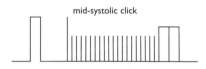

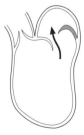

Cusp flails giving pansystolic regurgitation

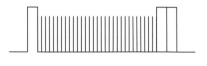

Aortic stenosis
- plateau pulse—narrow pulse pressure
- JVP only raised if heart failure
- LV_{++} systolic thrill
- soft a_2 with paradoxical split ($\pm$ ejection click)
- harsh mid systolic murmur, apex and base, radiating to carotids
    - note discrepancy of forceful apex and feeble arterial pulse
    - the longer the murmur, the tighter the stenosis. Loudness does not necessarily imply severity

Aortic incompetence
- water-hammer pulse—wide pulse pressure. Pulse visible in carotids
- JVP only raised if heart failure
- LV_{++} with dilation
- (ejection click)
- early diastolic murmur base $\rightarrow$ lower sternum (also ejection systolic murmur from increased flow)
    - (sometimes Austin Flint murmur—see below)
    - heard best with patient leaning forward, in expiration
    - the longer the murmur, the more severe the regurgitation

Tricuspid incompetence
- JVP large V wave
- RV_{++}, no thrill
- soft pansystolic murmur at maximal tricuspid area
- increases on inspiration

Austin Flint murmur
- mid diastolic murmur (like mitral stenosis) in aortic incompetence due to regurgitant stream of blood on anterior cusp mitral valve

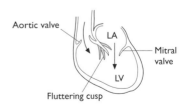

Aortic valve

LA

Mitral valve

LV

Fluttering cusp

Graham Steell murmur

- pulmonary early diastolic murmur (functional pulmonary incompetence) in mitral stenosis or other causes of pulmonary hypertension

Atrial septal defect

- JVP only raised if failure or tricuspid incompetence
- RV_{++} LVo
- widely fixed split-second sound
- pulmonary systolic murmur (tricuspid diastolic flow murmur)

Ventricular septal defect

- RV_+ LV_+
- Pansystolic murmur on left sternal edge (loud if small defect!)

Patent ductus arteriosus

- systolic $\rightarrow$ diastolic 'machinery' or continuous murmur below left clavicle

Metal prosthetic valves

- loud clicks with short flow murmur
  - aortic systolic
  - mitral diastolic
- need anticoagulation

Tissue prosthetic valves

- porcine xenograft or human homograft
- tend to fibrose after 7–10 years, leading to stenosis and incompetence
- may not require anticoagulation

Pericardial rub

- scratchy, superficial noise heard in systole and diastole
- brought out by stethoscope pressure, and sometimes variable with respiration

Infectious endocarditis (diagnosis made from blood cultures)

- febrile, unwell, anaemia
- clubbing
- splinter haemorrhages
- Osler's nodes
- cardiac murmur
- splenomegaly
- haematuria

Rheumatic fever

- flitting arthralgia
- erythema nodosum or erythema marginatum
- tachycardia
- murmurs
- *Sydenham's chorea* (irregular, uncontrollable jerks of limbs, tongue)

Clues to diagnosis from facial appearance

- *Down's syndrome* from 21 trisomy — ventricular septal defect
  — patent ductus arteriosus
- *thyrotoxicosis* — atrial fibrillation
- *myxoedema* from hypothyroid — cardiomyopathy
- dusky, congested face — *superior vena cava obstruction*
- red cheeks in infra-orbital region in mitral facies from mitral stenosis

Clues to diagnosis from general appearance

- *Turner's syndrome* from sex chromosomes X0
  - female, short stature, web of neck
  - coarctation of aorta
- *Marfan's syndrome*
  - tall patient with long, thin fingers
  - aortic regurgitation

Peripheral arteries

○ **Feel all peripheral pulses** (Fig. 3.4). Lower-limb pulses are usually felt after examining the abdomen.

Diminished or absent pulses suggest *arterial stenosis* or *occlusion*.

The lower-limb pulses are particularly important if there is a history of *intermittent claudication*.

Auscultation of the carotid and femoral vessels is useful if there is a suspicion these arteries are stenosed. A bruit is heard if the stenosis causes turbulent flow.

Coarctation of the aorta delays the femoral pulse after the radial pulse.

Peripheral vascular disease

— white or blue discoloration
— ulcers with little granulation tissue and slow healing
— shiny skin, loss of hairs, thickened dystrophic nails
— absent pulses
— Buerger's test of severity of arterial insufficiency
    — loss of autoregulation of blood flow
    — patient lying supine, lift leg up to 45° — positive test: pallor of foot; venous guttering
    — hang legs over side of bed: note time to capillary and venous filling; reactive hyperaemia; subsequent cyanosis

Diabetes, when present, also signs from **neuropathy**:
— dry skin with thickened epidermis
— callus from increased foot pressure over abnormal sites, e.g. under tarsal heads in mid-foot, secondary to motor neuropathy and change in distribution of weight (Plate 4f)
— absent ankle reflexes
— decreased sensation

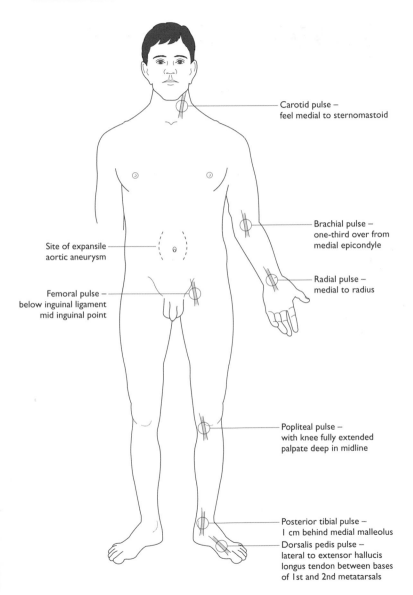

Carotid pulse –
feel medial to sternomastoid

Brachial pulse –
one-third over from
medial epicondyle

Radial pulse –
medial to radius

Site of expansile
aortic aneurysm

Femoral pulse –
below inguinal ligament
mid inguinal point

Popliteal pulse –
with knee fully extended
palpate deep in midline

Posterior tibial pulse –
1 cm behind medial malleolus

Dorsalis pedis pulse –
lateral to extensor hallucis
longus tendon between bases
of 1st and 2nd metatarsals

Fig. 3.4 Sites of peripheral pulses.

Aortic aneurysm

- central abdominal pulsation visible or palpable
- need to distinguish from normal, palpable aorta in midline in thin people
    - aortic aneurysm is expansible to each side as well as forwards
    - a bruit may be audible
    - associated with femoral and popliteal artery aneurysms

Varicose veins

O Varicose veins and herniae (see p. 95) are examined **when the patient is standing**, possibly at the end of the whole examination at the same time as the gait (see p. 45).

> Majority are associated with incompetent valves in the long saphenous vein or short saphenous vein.

> Long saphenous—from femoral vein in groin to medial side of lower leg.

> Short saphenous—from popliteal fossa to back of calf and lateral malleolus.

O **Observe:**
- swelling
- pigmentation ⎤
- eczema ⎦ indicate chronic venous insufficiency
- inflammation—suggests thrombophlebitis

O **Palpate:**
- soft or hard (thrombosed)
- tender—thrombophlebitis
- cough impulse—implies incompetent valves

Incompetent valves can be confirmed by the **Trendelenburg test**:

- Elevate leg to empty veins.
- Occlude long saphenous vein with a tourniquet around upper thigh.
- Stand patient up.
- If veins fill rapidly, this indicates incompetent thigh perforators below the tourniquet.

- If, after release of tourniquet, veins fill rapidly, this indicates incompetent saphenofemoral junction.

If veins fill immediately on standing, then incompetent valves are in thigh or calf, so do the **Perthes test**:

- As for Trendelenburg, but on standing let some blood enter veins by temporary release of groin pressure.
- Ask patient to stand up and down on toes.
- Veins become less tense if:
  - muscle pump is satisfactory
  - perforating calf veins are patent with competent valves

System-oriented examination

'Examine the cardiovascular system'

- hands—splinter haemorrhages
- radial pulse—rate, rhythm, waveform, volume, state of artery
- waveform and volume best examined at the brachial or carotid artery
- *'I would normally measure the blood pressure now; would you like me to do so?'*
- eyes—anaemia
- tongue—central cyanosis
- JVP—height, waveform
- apex beat—site, character
- auscultate—at apex (with thumb on carotid artery for timing)
  - heart sounds
  - added sounds
  - murmurs
  - in neck over carotid artery—each area of precordium with diaphragm
    - aortic incompetence—lean forward in full expiration with diaphragm
    - mitral stenosis—lie patient on left side and listen at apex with bell
- *'I would normally now listen to the bases for crepitations, examine for hepatomegaly, peripheral oedema and peripheral pulses. Would you like me to do so?'*

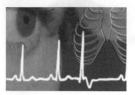

CHAPTER 4

Examination of the Chest

General inspection

○ **Examine the patient for:**
- end of bed for signs of respiratory distress — use of accessory muscles, on oxygen therapy, inspect sputum pot
- **nicotine** on fingers
- **clubbing**: respiratory causes include:
  carcinoma of bronchus
  mesothelioma
  bronchiectasis
  lung abscess
  empyema
  fibrosing alveolitis
- **evidence of respiratory failure**:
  - **hypoxia**: central cyanosis
  - **hypercapnia**: drowsiness, confusion, papilloedema, warm hands, bounding pulse, dilated veins, coarse tremor/flap
- **respiratory rate**: count per minute
- **pattern of respiration: Cheyne–Stokes**:
  - alternating hyperventilation and apnoea
  - severe increased intracranial pressure
  - left ventricular failure
  - high altitude
- **obstructive airways disease**:
  - pursed-lip breathing:
    - expiration against partially closed lips
    - chronic obstructive airways disease to delayed closure of bronchioles

- use of accessory muscles:

sternomastoids

strap muscles and platysmus

- **wheezing**
- **stridor**: partial obstruction of major airway
- **hoarse voice**:

abnormal vocal cords

or *recurrent laryngeal palsy*

First examine the front of the chest fully and then similarly examine the back of the chest.

Inspection of the chest

O **Rest the patient comfortably in the bed at 45°**
  - distended neck, puffy blue face and arms
  - superior mediastinal obstruction
O **Inspect the shape of the chest**
  - asymmetry: diminution of one side

    lung collapse

    fibrosis
  - deformity: check spine

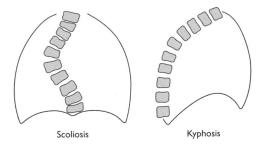

Scoliosis   Kyphosis

- pectus excavatum: sunken sternum
- **obstructive airways disease**
  - barrel chest: lower costal recession on deep inspiration. Cricoid cartilage close to sternal notch. Chest appears to be fixed in inspiration

Palpation

- **Check mediastinum position**
  - **trachea**—check position: palpate with a single finger in the midline and determine if it slips preferentially to one side or the other.

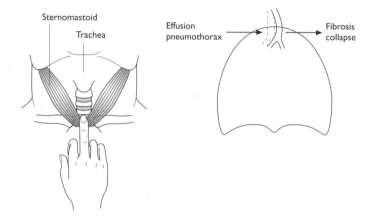

- **Lymph nodes,** supraclavicular fossae/axillae—*tuberculosis, lymphoma, cancer of the bronchus*
- **Apex beat** may be displaced because of enlarged heart and not a shift in the mediastinum.
- **Unequal movement of chest.**
  - Look from the end of the bed.
  - Classic method of palpation:
    - extend your fingers—anchor fingertips far laterally around chest wall so your extended thumbs meet in midline
    - on inspiration, assess whether asymmetrical movement of thumbs from midline

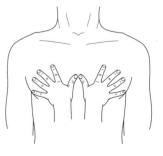

— Alternative method of palpation:
  — lay a hand comfortably on either side of the chest and, using these as a gauge, assess if there is diminution of movement on one side during inspiration

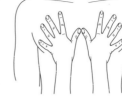

N.B. Diminution of movement on one side indicates pathology on that side.

Percussion

O Percuss with the middle finger of one hand against the middle phalanx of the middle finger of the other, laid flat on the chest. The finger should strike at right angles.

O **Percuss both sides of the chest for resonance**, at top, middle and lower segments. Compare sides, and if different also compare the front and back of chest.

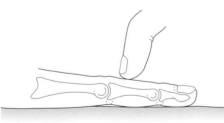

Chest wall

O If a dull area exists, map out its limits by percussing from a resonant to the dull area.

O Percuss the level of the diaphragm from above downwards.

Increased resonance may occur in:

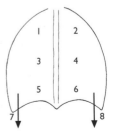

> — *pneumothorax*
> — *emphysema*

Decreased resonance may occur in:

> — *effusion*: very dull—sometimes called stony dullness
> — *solid lung*
>> — consolidation
>> — collapse
>> — abscess

— neoplasm

Remember the surface markings of the lungs when percussing.

Thus, the lower lobe predominates posteriorly and the upper lobe predominates anteriorly (Fig. 4.1).

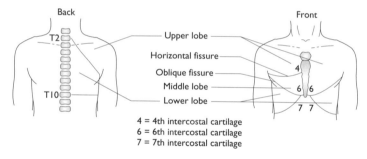

4 = 4th intercostal cartilage
6 = 6th intercostal cartilage
7 = 7th intercostal cartilage

Fig. 4.1 Percuss the diaphragm from above downwards. These markings are at full inspiration. Under normal examination conditions the hepatic dullness extends to the fifth intercostal cartilage.

Auscultation

- **Before listening, ask patient to cough up any sputum** which may provide noises for bronchi.
- Use the bell of the stethoscope and listen at the top, middle and bottom of both sides of the chest, and then in the axilla.

Ask the patient to breathe through his mouth moderately deeply. It helps to demonstrate this yourself.

The stethoscope diaphragm is less effective if the patient is thin with prominent ribs or if the chest is hairy.

O **Listen for breath sounds,** comparing both sides (Fig. 4.2):
  — **vesicular:** normal breath sounds

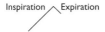

  — **bronchial:** patent bronchi plus conducting tissue

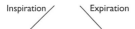

  — sounds similar to sounds with stethoscope over trachea
      consolidation (usually pneumonia)
      neoplasm
      fibrosis
      abscess
  not collapse, effusion (except occasionally at surface)
  — **diminution**: indicates either no air movement (e.g. obstructed bronchus) or air or fluid preventing sound conduction
      effusion
      pneumothorax
      emphysema
      collapse

O **Listen for added sounds,** and note if inspiratory or expiratory:
  — **pleural rub**: caused by *pleurisy* (inflammation due to infection or infarction), but make sure it does not come from friction of skin or hairs against stethoscope
  — **rhonchi or wheezing**: constricted air passages giving dry tubular sounds, often maximal on expiration
  — **râles or crepitations** or crackles:
      — fine—*heart failure* or *alveolitis*
      — medium—*infection*

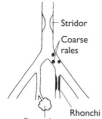

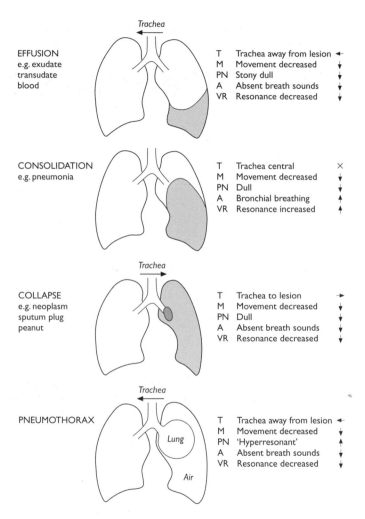

Fig. 4.2 Auscultation.

— coarse—air bubbling through fluid in larger bronchioles, e.g. *bronchiectasis*. If relieved by coughing, suggests from bronchioles

Vocal resonance

Normally only done if pathology is suspected, but you must practise to become familiar with normal resonance.

O **Ask the patient to repeat '99'** whilst listening to chest in the same areas as auscultation. The sounds are louder over areas of consolidation. Compare both sides.

At the surface of an *effusion* the words '99' take on a bleating character like a goat, which is called **aegophony**. If vocal resonance is gross, **whispering pectoriloquy** can be elicited by asking the patient to whisper: '1, 2, 3, 4'.

N.B. Vocal fremitus, breath sounds and vocal resonance all depend on the same criteria and vary together.

To determine further clues check:
— chest movement asymmetry
— mediastinum displacement
— percussion

Sputum

Examination of the sputum is unpleasant but important.

O Look for:
— **quantity** (increased grossly in bronchiectasis)
— **consistency** (if all mucus it may be saliva)
— **colour** (in yellow or green it may be infected)
— **blood** – *cancer, tuberculosis, embolus*

Ideally the sputum should be examined under the microscope for:
— bacteria
— pus cells
— eosinophils
— plugs
— asbestos

Functional result

○ Make an assessment of the functional result:
  — **History.** How far can the patient walk, etc.
  — **Examination**:
    — $Po_2\downarrow$: central cyanosis
      confusion
    — $Pco_2\uparrow$: peripheral signs — warm periphery
                                       — dilated veins
                                       — bounding pulse
                                       — flapping tremor
      central signs   — drowsy
                       — papilloedema
                       — small pupils
  — check by arterial blood gases
  — **Tests** (usually of obstructive airways disease):
    — **At the bedside**: blowing out a lighted match about 15 cm from the mouth and with the mouth wide open is easy as long as your peak flow is above approximately 80 l/min (normal 300–500 l/min).
    — **Expiration time**: an assessment of airways obstruction can be made by timing the period of full expiration through wide-open mouth following a deep breath. This should be less than 2 seconds when normal.
    — **Chest expansion**: expansion from full inspiration to full expiration should be more than 5cm. Reduced if hyperinflation of the chest is due to chronic obstructive airways disease.
    — **Peak flow meter**: a measure of airways obstruction is the peak rate of flow of air out of the lungs. A record is made using a machine. Normal 300–500 l/min.

Summary of common illnesses

Asthma

  — patient distressed, tachypnoeic, unable to talk easily
  — wheeze on expiration audible or by auscultation

- overinflated chest with hyperresonance
- if central cyanosis: critically ill, artificial ventilation?
- pulsus paradoxus (may be normal between attacks)
- often due to atopy
  - enquire about exposure to antigens:
    - house dust mite
    - cats or dogs

Obstructive airways disease (chronic)

- barrel chest
- accessory muscles of respiration in use
- hyperresonance
- depressed diaphragm—indrawing lower costal margin on inspiration
- diminished breath sounds:
  - **blue bloater**:
    central cyanosis
    signs of carbon dioxide retention
    obese
    not dyspnoeic
    ankle oedema: may or may not have right heart failure
  - **pink puffer**:
    not cyanosed
    no carbon dioxide retention
    thin
    dyspnoeic
    no oedema

Bronchiectasis

- clubbing
- constant green/yellow phlegm
- coarse râles over affected area

Allergic alveolitis

- clubbing
- fine, unexplained râles, widespread over bases

System-oriented examination

'Examine the respiration system'

- hands: clubbing, signs of increased carbon dioxide (warm hands, bounding pulse, coarse tremor)
- tongue: central cyanosis
- trachea
- supraclavicular nodes
- inspection
  - shape of chest
  - chest movements
  - respiration rate/distress
- palpation: unequal movement of chest using hands
- percussion: upper segments (L, R), middle (L, R) and lower segments (L, R)
- auscultation:
  - breath sounds
  - added sounds: crepitations, bronchospasm, pleural rub, stridor (vocal fremitus)
- if obstructive airways disease:
  - expiration time (see p. 84)

CHAPTER 5

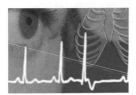

Examination of the Abdomen

General inspection

O Look for signs of:

- **chronic liver disease:**
  - *clubbing*
  - *leukonychia*
  - *palmar erythema*
  - *telangiectasia* on face
  - *icterus* (Plate 1e)
  - *spider naevi* (Plate 1f)
  - *gynaecomastia*
  - *alcohol abuse*
    - *Dupuytren's contracture* (Plate 4c)
    - *parotid enlargement*
    - *testicular atrophy*

Spider naevus: a small collection of capillaries fed by a central arteriole

- **liver failure:**
  - *liver flap*
  - *foetor hepaticus*
  - *confusion*

    Signs of chronic liver disease are usually obvious, but we are all allowed up to six spider naevi (particularly if pregnant!).

- **anaemia**—look at conjunctiva, tongue
- **iron deficiency:**
  - *koilonychia* (Plate 2d)
  - *smooth tongue*
  - *angular stomatitis*—can be from ill-fitting dentures or edentulous state
- **B$_{12}$ or folate deficiency**—'beef steak' or smooth tongue

○ **Look at lips:**
 — pale — examine conjunctivae for anaemia
    — Brown freckles — *Peutz–Jeghers syndrome* — polyps in small
      bowel can bleed, intussuscept or become malignant.
    — Telangiectasia — *Osler–Weber–Rendu syndrome* — gastroin-
      testinal telangiectasia can bleed.
○ **Look at mouth:**
 — **dry tongue** — 'dehydration' or mouth-breathing
      If patient seems dehydrated, lift fold of skin on neck. Skin
      remains raised with dehydration and old age.
 — central cyanosis in chronic liver disease from pulmonary arteriovenous shunting
 — *Candida* — red tongue, white patches on palate
 — *gingivitis*
 — ulcers
    — Crohn's disease, ulcerative colitis
    — aphthous with coeliac disease
 — teeth
 — breath — *ketosis*, *ethanol*, *foetor hepaticus* and *uraemia*
○ **Palpate for nodes** behind the left sternoclavicular joint.

A hard node felt behind the
left sternoclavicular joint may
be a **Virchow's node** and
suggests an abdominal neoplasm spread by lymphatics via
the thoracic duct.

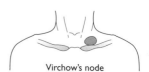

Virchow's node

Inspection of the abdomen

○ **Lie the patient flat** (one pillow) with arms by his sides.
○ **Expose the abdomen** from chest margin to groin.

**In an exam, stand back to look at the abdomen, so the examiner
is impressed you are inspecting before palpating!**
○ **Look for:**
 — skin — striae: pink in *Cushing's syndrome*

- body hair
- nodules
- surgical scars
- swelling—central or flank
    - symmetrical or asymmetrical. May be due to:
        - flatus
        - faeces
        - fetus
        - fat
        - fluid (ascites, ovarian cyst)
- movement: on respiration
- peristalsis: may be visible in thin normal person
- pulsation
- hernia
- dilated veins—flow of blood in vein (Fig. 5.1) is:

    - **superior**: due to inferior vena cava obstruction
    - **inferior**: due to superior vena cava obstruction
    - **radiating from navel**: due to portal vein hypertension

Describe findings using these descriptions:

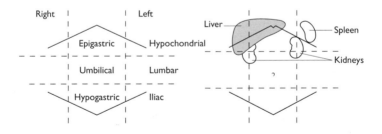

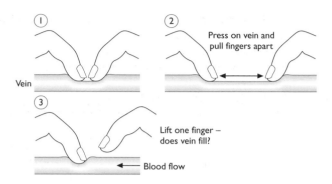

Fig. 5.1 William Harvey's method of checking vein filling.

Palpation of the abdomen

○ **Palpate the groins** for enlarged lymph nodes. (If you don't do it now, you may forget later!)

   Most people have small, shotty nodes. Most enlarged tender nodes arise from infection in legs or feet.

   If large nodes, palpate spleen carefully—lymphoma or leukaemia.

○ **Before you feel abdomen**:
   — **Ask**: 'Is your tummy painful anywhere? Tell me if I hurt you.'
   — **Have warm hands**, and the patient lying flat.
   — **Lightly palpate each quadrant first**, starting away from the site of pain or tenderness. The hand should be flat on the abdomen and feel by flexing fingers at the metacarpophalangeal joints. Be gentle.
   — **Look at the patient's face** to see if palpation is hurting him.
   — **Deep palpation**. If there is no evidence of distress palpate the abdomen in the same manner but deeper.

      Tenderness may be superficial, deep or rebound.

      Rebound tenderness from movement of inflamed viscera of peritonitis against parietal peritoneum. First percuss abdomen lightly, then move vigorously. If no pain, can proceed to deep palpation with sudden removal of hand.

Guarding may be noted during palpation. This is a voluntary muscle spasm to protect from pain.

Rigidity. Fixed, tense abdominal muscles from reflex involuntary spasm. Occurs in generalized peritonitis.

Palpation of the organs

Liver

- **Palpate** with fingers flexed at metacarpophalangeal joints, using side of forefinger parallel with liver, with the patient breathing moderately deeply. Start about 10 cm below the costal margin and work up towards the ribs.
- **Describe position of liver edge** in centimetres below the costal margin of the mid clavicular line. Feel surface of enlarged liver and edge for:
  - **texture**
  - **regular/irregular edge**
  - **tender**
  - **pulsatile** (in tricuspid incompetence)
- **Percuss the upper and lower borders of liver** after palpation to confirm findings.

  If the liver is not felt and the right hypochondrium is dull, the liver may extend to the hypogastrium! Palpate lower down.
- If the liver is large, describe:

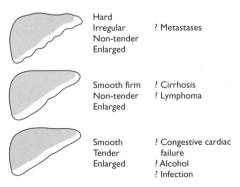

Hard
Irregular   ? Metastases
Non-tender
Enlarged

Smooth firm   ? Cirrhosis
Non-tender   ? Lymphoma
Enlarged

Smooth   ? Congestive cardiac
Tender   failure
Enlarged   ? Alcohol
                     ? Infection

If large, remember to feel for the spleen.

Spleen

- As for the liver, **palpate** 10 cm beneath the costal margin in the hypochondrium, working up to ribs.
- **Ask the patient to take a deep breath**, to bring the spleen down so it can be palpated.
- If the spleen is not palpable, **percuss** area for splenic dullness—the spleen can be enlarged to the hypogastrium!

    If a slightly enlarged spleen is suspected, lie the patient on the right side with the left arm hanging loosely in front and again feel on deep inspiration.

- **Check** characteristics of the spleen:
    - **site**
    - **shape (?notch)**
    - **cannot get above it**
    - **moves on respiration**
    - **dull to percussion**
- Describe as for liver.

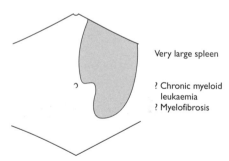

Very large spleen

? Chronic myeloid
   leukaemia
? Myelofibrosis

Kidneys

- **Palpate bimanually.**
- **Push up with left hand in renal angle** and feel kidney anteriorly with right hand.
- **Ask the patient to take a deep breath** to bring kidneys between hands.

    Tenderness is common over the kidneys if there is infection. A large kidney may indicate a *tumour*, *polycystic disease* or *hydronephrosis*.

Masses

o **Carefully palpate the whole of the abdomen.** If a mass is found, describe:
  - **site**
  - **size**
  - **shape**
  - **consistency**—faeces may be indented by pressure
  - **fixation or mobility**—does it move on respiration?
  - **tender**
  - **pulsatile**—transmitted pulsation from aorta or pulsatile swelling
  - **dull to percussion**—particularly important to determine if bowel is in front of mass
  - **does it alter after defaecation or micturition?**

Aorta

o **Palpate in the midline above the umbilicus** for a pulsatile mass. If easily palpated, suspect aortic aneurysm and proceed to ultrasonography in males over 50 and women over 60 years.
  - may be normal aorta in a thin person
  - unfolded aorta
  - aneurysm

Percussion

Dullness on percussion:
  - ascites—free fluid
  - an organ, e.g. liver, spleen
  - tumour, e.g. *large ovarian cyst*
o **Percuss liver, speen and kidneys after palpation of each organ.**
o **Percuss any suspected mass.**

  The midline of the abdomen should be resonant—if not, think of *gastric neoplasm*, *omental secondaries*, *enlarged bladder*, *ovarian cyst*, *pregnancy*.

O   If there is generalized swelling of the abdomen, lie the patient on one side and mark the upper level of dullness. Roll the patient to the other side and see if the level shifts. This is called **shifting dullness.**

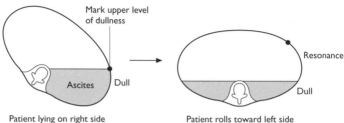

Patient lying on right side   Patient rolls toward left side

Auscultation

Bowel sounds

O   Listen over the abdomen with the diaphragm of the stethoscope.

Obstruction of the bowel gives hyperactive 'tinkling' bowel sounds.

Paralytic ileus or *generalized peritonitis* give complete absence of bowel sounds.

O   Listen for hepatic bruits in patients with liver disease:
– *primary liver cell cancer*
– *alcoholic hepatitis*
– *acquired arteriovenous shunts* from biopsy or trauma

Arterial bruits

If appropriate from the history or examination (e.g. hypertension), listen for bruits over the renal or femoral arteries. Renal arteries are sometimes best heard over the back.

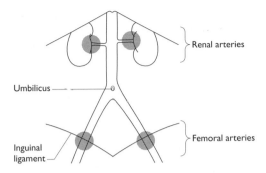

Renal artery stenosis may be the cause of hypertension.

Patients with *intermittent claudication* may have flow bruits over the femoral arteries from narrowing, e.g. *atheroma*.

Herniae

o **Establish the appropriate anatomical landmarks**—pubic symphysis, anterior superior iliac spine, femoral artery.

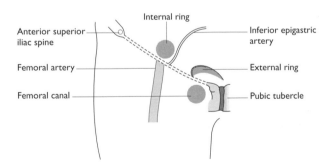

o **Examine the patient standing and ask him to cough**—enlargement of a groin swelling suggests a hernia.

Indirect (oblique) inguinal hernia: swelling reduced to

internal inguinal ring by pressure on contents of hernial sac and then controlled by pressure over the internal ring when patient asked to cough. If hand is then removed, **impulse passes medially towards external ring and is palpable above the pubic tubercle**.

Direct inguinal hernia: impulse in a forward direction mainly above groin crease **medial to femoral artery** and swelling not controlled by pressure over internal ring.

Femoral hernia: swelling fills out the groin crease medial to the femoral artery.

Examination of genitals

O **Ask in a sensitive way** before you proceed, e.g. 'I should briefly examine you down below. Is that all right?'

O **In the male, palpate the scrotum** for the testes and epididymes. It is rarely necessary to examine the penis.

Tender and enlarged testes may occur with *orchitis* or *torsion of the testis*.

A **large, hard, painless testis** suggests *cancer*.

A **large, soft swelling which transilluminates** suggests *hydrocele* or an *epididymal cyst*. A hydrocele surrounds the testis; an epididymal cyst lies behind the testis.

Balanitis (inflamed glans of penis) should remind the examiner to check for diabetes.

Per rectum examination

Never perform a rectal examination without permission from the houseman or registrar or without a chaperone for female patients.

O Tell the patient at each stage what you are going to do.

O Lie the patient on the left side with knees flexed to the chest.

O Say: 'I am going to put a finger into your back passage'.

O Inspect anus for haemorrhoids and fissures.

O With lubricant on glove, gently insert forefinger into rectum. Feel the tone of the sphincter, size and character of the prostate and any lateral masses. If appropriate, proceed to proctoscopy.

o Test stool on your glove for occult blood.

Per vaginam examination

Never perform a vaginal examination without a chaperone, female if possible, and only on the direction of a qualified instructor.

o Tell the patient at each stage what you are going to do.
o Lie the patient on her left side as for per rectum examination (although some physicians prefer patient lying on her back with hips flexed and abducted).
o Inspect the external genitalia.
o With lubricant on glove insert one finger into vagina and then a second finger if there is room.
o Palpate the cervix.
o Examine for position and enlargement of uterus, tenderness of appendages and masses.
o Check for discharge by observing glove.

Summary of common illnesses

Cirrhosis
- white nails
- clubbing
- liver palms
- spider naevi
- jaundice
- firm liver

Portal hypertension
- splenomegaly
- ascites
- caput medusa

Hepatic encephalopathy

- liver flap
- drowsy
- constructional apraxia (cannot draw five-pointed star)
- musty foetor

'Dehydration' (water and salt loss)

- dry skin
- veins collapsed
- diminished skin turgor — pinched fold of skin remains raised
- tongue dry
- eyes sunken
- blood pressure low with postural drop

Intestinal obstruction

- patient 'dehydrated' if he has been vomiting
- abdomen centrally swelling
- visible peristalsis
- not tender (unless inflammation, or some other pathology)
- resonant to percussion
- loud 'tinkling' bowel sounds

Pyloric stenosis

- upper abdomen swelling
- may have 'succussion splash' on shaking abdomen
- otherwise like intestinal obstruction

Appendicitis

- slight fever
- deep tenderness right iliac fossa or per rectum
- otherwise little to find unless has spread to peritonitis

Peritonitis

- lies still
- abdomen
  - does not move on respiration

- rigid on palpation (guarding)
- tender, particularly on removing fingers rapidly (rebound tenderness)
- absent bowel sounds

Cholecystitis
- tender right hypochondrium, particularly on breathing in (Murphy's sign—tender gallbladder descends on inspiration to touch your palpating hand)

Jaundice and palpable gallbladder
- obstruction is not due to gallstones, but from another obstruction such as a neoplasm of the pancreas (Courvoisier's law). Gallstones have usually caused a fibrosed gallbladder which cannot dilate from back-pressure from gallstones in common bile duct

Enlarged spleen
- infective, e.g. *septicaemia* or *subacute bacterial endocarditis*
- portal hypertension, e.g. *cirrhosis*
- *lymphoma*, leukaemia and other haematological diseases
- autoimmune, e.g. systemic lupus, Felty's syndrome

System-oriented examination
'Examine the abdomen'
- hands: clubbing, liver flap, Dupuytren's contracture
- eyes: jaundice, anaemia
- tongue: foetor, smooth
- neck: Virchow's lymph node
- chest: spider naevi, gynaecomastia
- palpate inguinal lymph nodes briefly
- inspect abdomen asymmetry, movement, pulsation, swelling
- enquire whether pain or tenderness
- palpate four quadrants for masses: note abdominal tenderness, guarding, rigidity

- palpate liver, kidneys, spleen, aortic aneurysm
- ascites: test for shifting dullness
- auscultate bowel sounds, arterial or liver bruits
- examine for hernia: ask patient to cough. Stand patient up if a hernia is a possibility
- enquire whether appropriate:
    - to examine vulva/testes
    - to do rectal examination

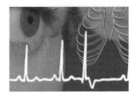

CHAPTER 6

Examination of the Mental State

Introduction

Examination of the mental state is necessary in all patients, not just those seen in psychiatric settings. The main headings are:

- **appearance and behaviour**
- **mood**
- **speech** — rate, form, content
- **thinking** — form, content
- **abnormal beliefs** — odd ideas and delusions
- **abnormal perceptions** — hallucinations and illusions
- **cognitive function** — concentration, orientation, memory, reasoning
- **understanding of condition**

The distinction between history and examination becomes blurred when examining disordered mental states.

Much of the examination is done by careful observation whilst taking the history, and then supplemented with additional questions afterwards (see pp. 16–17 for mental state history, pp. 112–117 for examination).

If there is difficulty obtaining a clear history or if the patient appears distressed, it is particularly important to examine the mental state.

General rules

- ○ Be non-judgemental.
- ○ Be alert to phenomenon that are observed.
- ○ Do not jump to conclusions about what the patient is saying.
- ○ Clarify with gentle enquiry:
    - — **'Can you tell me more about that?'**

- 'Can you give me a recent example?'
- 'When did that last happen?'
- 'What did you do about it?'
- 'How often/how long have you experienced that?'

Appearance and behaviour (observation)

O Describe in simple terms:
  - unkempt appearance
  - bewildered, agitated, restless, aggressive, tearful, sullen:
    - appropriate to setting?
    - reduced activity in *depression*
    - overactive and intrusive in *mania*
    - tense and reassurance seeking with *anxiety*
  - able to respond to questions
  - evidence of responding to hallucinations
  - smell of alcohol
  - evidence of drug misuse (e.g. needle marks)

Mood (part observation, part enquiry)

> Mood is a subjective state and is mainly judged by the impression conveyed during the history, although examination gives further clues.

O Ask:
  - 'How have your spirits been recently?'
  - 'Have you been feeling your normal self?'
  - 'Is this how you normally feel?'

    > Depressed—depression disorder or an adjustment reaction (see questions on p. 16)
    > Elevated—manic disorder or intoxication, e.g. ethanol, drugs, delirium.
    > Anxious—anxiety disorder or reaction to situation.
    > Angry—delirium or reaction to situation.
    > Flat—depressed or no emotional rapport, i.e. *schizophrenia*.

O If evidence for depression, worry, agitation, irritability—record current nature and severity.
  - if depressed, ask

- 'How bad has it been?'
- 'Have you ever thought of suicide?'
- 'Have you seriously considered taking your life?'

O Also ask for nurses' and relatives' comments.

Speech (observation)

Describe speech in simple terms and record verbatim typical remarks.

O **Rate:**
  - fast in *mania*
  - slow in *depression*
O **Form:**
  - are there abnormalities of grammar or flow? Record examples
    Disordered thought processes can occur in *schizophrenia, mania, acute organic states, dementia*.
  - are there abnormal sequences of words?
    - non-sequiters with disordered logic in *schizophrenia*—'word jumble'
    - loosely connected topics in *mania*—'flight of ideas'
O **Content** (observations, elaborate with enquiry):
  - 'You said you . . . , tell me more about that'
  - 'When you feel sad, what goes through your mind?'

Thinking (form and content—largely inferred from speech)

O Record patient's main thoughts or preoccupations:
  - negative pessimistic in *depression*—ask about suicidal intentions
  - grandiose in *mania*
  - catastrophizing in *anxiety*
    Obsessions—intrusive thoughts or repetitious behaviours which the patient cannot resist although he knows they are not sensible.
  - perseveration—repetition of a word or phrase. Can occur in *anxiety, depression, mania, delirium* or *dementia*

Abnormal beliefs (odd ideas and delusions)

O Ask to describe; be non-judgemental.

○ Ask why he thinks that—may reveal psychotic thoughts or hallucinations.

> **Delusions** are fixed, false beliefs without reasonable evidence, e.g. I've got AIDS/cancer.

— 'Did it ever seem to you that people were talking about you?'
— 'Have you ever received special messages from the television, radio or newspaper?'
— 'Do people seem to be going out of their way to get at you?'
— 'Have you ever felt that you were especially important in some way or that you had special powers?'
— 'Do you ever feel you have committed a crime or done something terrible for which you should be punished?'

Abnormal perceptions (hallucinations and illusions — usually apparent from history)

○ Ask—'Have you had any unusual experiences recently?'
— 'Do they seem as if they are in the real world or as if they are 'inside' your head?'

> **Hallucinations** are false perceptions without a stimulus (e.g. pink elephants—experienced as real).
>
> — They can occur in any sensory modality.
> — Visual hallucinations are suggestive of an organic state.
> — Third person ('he' or 'she') auditory hallucinations are suggestive of *schizophrenia*.
>> — 'Do you ever hear things that other people can't hear such as the voices of people talking?'
>> — 'Do you ever have visions or see things that other people can't see?'
>> — 'Do you ever have strange sensations in your body or skin?'
>
> **Illusions** are misinterpreted perceptions (e.g. he thinks you are a policeman). They are common in acute organic states (*psychosis*).

Cognitive functioning (observations supplemented by specific enquiry)

O **Impairment of concentration** can occur in:
   - *depression*
   - *anxiety states*
   - *dementia*
   - *confusional state*

O **Orientation, thought processes, memory and logic.** These aspects must be tested as part of examination of the mental state (see Examination of the nervous system, p. 112).

Understanding of condition

O **'What do you think is wrong with you?'**
   - **'Is there any illness that you are particularly worried about?'**
   - **'What treatment do you feel is appropriate?'**
   - **'Are there any treatments you are frightened of?'**

      It is important to ask all patients these questions. If the patient lacks insight into abnormal beliefs or behaviour, this suggests a psychotic illness.

General history and examination

Mental illness can be the presentation of a physical illness and a full history and examination should be done in all patients.

   Physical illnesses that masquerade as mental illnesses include:
   - *hypothyroid, hyperthyroid*
   - *hypercalcaemia, hypokalaemia, hypomagnesaemia* or *hyponatraemia*
   - *cerebral tumour*
   - *other causes of increased intracranial pressure*
   - *chronic, occult infection*
   - *drugs*
   - *porphyria*

It is arguable that all mental illness arises from a physical imbalance of transmitters/receptor function in the brain, and the division of illness into physical and mental is spurious. In any case, all patients, whatever the nature of their illness, should be treated non-judgementally and with respect.

Problem patients

Angry patients

- Inordinate anger is often symptomatic of another problem.
- Assess whether the grievance is justified and whether it can be resolved.
- 'Is there anything else that is upsetting you?'
- If the antagonism is directed against you, enquire whether the patient would prefer to see somebody else.

Aggressive patients

- Do not take risks (have help nearby).
- Ensure patient does not have a weapon.
- Determine orientation and whether intoxicated or deluded.
- Fear often underlines aggression—what is the fear?

Tearful patients

- If a patient starts to weep, be calm and gently sympathetic.
- When less tearful, enquire why they are upset. If you can find out reason:
    - it may help rapport
    - it may allow resolution of the problem

Suicidal patients

- Assess intent of recent attempt (if any):
    - planning and likelihood of discovery
    - perceived dangerousness of method
    - intention at time
- Assess current intent:
    - how likely to attempt suicide?
    - what does he want to happen?
    - what would increase/decrease risk?

Embarrassed patients

- Patients may not wish to talk about a distressing situation.
- It may help to reassure about confidentiality.
- If you think you know the problem, you can bring it up:
    - 'Is there a problem with money/sex/children, etc?'
- If the patient really does not want to talk about a problem, it is better to leave it and broach it later, possibly at another interview.

Talkative patients

Some patients go into irrelevant detail, digress and repeat themselves.

- Remind patient of time left and need to cover main points. Check what they are and proceed.
- Politely say 'Thank you. Please help me with some specific questions . . . ' and proceed to specific questions that require answers.

Nonsense history

- Occasionally you get nowhere—contradictory remarks, description of improbable events, perseveration or just silence and monosyllables.
- Change to other aspects of history, e.g. personal or family history, social circumstances.
- If these also do not help, proceed if feasible to examination. You may identify *dementia, evidence of drug abuse, hysteria* or some other illness which explains the problem.
- Essential to interview other informants (e.g. telephone a relative).

Summary of common illnesses

Depression

- low mood, tearfulness (not always present)
- lack of interest and self-care
- poor concentration
- negative thought content
- low self-esteem
- wakes up early
- depressed facies

- slow movements and speech
- weight loss
- negative speech content

Anxiety
- generally worried
- thought focuses on catastrophies
- cannot get to sleep
- tense lined face, furrowed brow
- sweaty palms
- shaky
- hyperventilation
- tachycardia

Anorexia nervosa
- thin, little body fat
- increased, fine body hair
- sees self as fat even if thin
- thoughts dominated by food

Bulimia nervosa
- often normal weight
- binges followed by self-induced vomiting
- thoughts dominated by food
- erosion of teeth from vomiting

Acute psychosis (schizophrenia, mania or depressive psychosis)
- alert and oriented
- normal activities disrupted
- unpredictable behaviour
- reports or behaves as if responding to hallucinations
- reports delusional beliefs

Schizophrenic psychosis
- illogical thought, even a disjointed 'word salad'
- auditory hallucinations (third person)

- delusions (especially concerning thoughts, e.g. broadcast)
- activity may be responding to hallucinations and delusions

Manic psychosis

- rapid speech with 'flight of ideas'
- overactive, cannot keep still
- normal activities disrupted
- overly cheerful or irritable
- stands close and is argumentative

Depressive psychosis

- depressed affect
- slow movements and speech
- negative thoughts and delusions, e.g. brain is rotting
- suicidal thoughts

Chronic schizophrenia

- alert and oriented
- unkempt
- odd rambling speech
- elaborate delusions
- mannerisms and odd gestures
- look for tardive dyskinesia (parkinsonian features from long-term neuroleptic treatment)

Delirium

- fluctuating level of concentration and orientation—worse at night
- fleeting delusions, often persecutory in nature
- evidence of toxicity (fever, etc.)

Intoxication (a type of delirium)

- smells of alcohol or glue
- needle marks
- impaired alertness and drowsy
- visual hallucinations

Dementia

- alert (unless also delirious)
- may be unkempt
- poor orientation in time and space
- cognitive function subnormal
    - poor short-term memory
    - cannot remember recent events
    - cannot remember and repeat series of numbers or an address
    - cannot explain proverbs
- paucity of thought and speech

Bereavement

- low mood and tearfulness when thinking of lost person
- may have somatic symptoms
- assess suicide risk (to join lost person)
- if excessively severe or prolonged (more than 6 months), may be considered 'pathological'

Somatization/hypochondriasis

- somatic symptoms (often pain, fatigue) with no organic disease
- assess for sign of depression
- determine patient's illness, fears or beliefs
- symptoms are main concern in *somatization*, fear of illness in *hypochondriasis*

CHAPTER 7

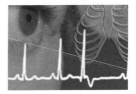

Examination of the Nervous System

Introduction

The goal of the examination is to answer three questions: (1) Does the patient have a neurological illness? (2) Where in the nervous system is the pathology located? (3) What is the pathology?

As always, the history is critical. The following features in the history can be informative:

- **onset**
    - abrupt — *vascular, mechanical*
    - seconds — *seizure*
    - minutes — *migraine*
    - hours — *infective, inflammatory*
    - days/weeks — *neoplasm* or *degenerative disorder*
- **duration**
    - brief episodes with recovery, e.g. *TIA, epilepsy, migraine, syncope*
    - longer episodes with recovery — *mechanical, obstruction or pressure*
    - demyelination, e.g. *multiple scelorsis*
- **frequency**
- **witness description** — particularly if the patient has episodic loss of consciousness or is confused.

The examination of the nervous system can be elaborated almost indefinitely. Of far greater importance is **to acquire the ability to conduct a thorough but comparatively rapid examination with confidence in the findings**. It is best to develop your own basic system for doing the examination and to perform it consistently. This will avoid omissions.

o **Adapt your examination to the situation.** The routine examination must be mastered but can be altered to fit the situation.

The examination of the nervous system is approached under the following headings:

o **Higher cerebral function.**
o **Cranial nerves.**
o **Motor.**
o **Coordination.**
o **Reflexes.**
o **Sensation.**
o **Gait and station.**

The nervous system cannot be examined in isolation.

Other points of relevance may include:
  - configuration of the skull and spine
  - neck stiffness
  - ear drums for otitis media
  - blood pressure
  - heart, e.g. arrhythmia, mitral stenosis
  - carotid arteries — palpation and bruit
  - neoplasms — breast, lung, abdominal
  - jaundice

Higher cerebral functions

Higher mental functions can only be properly assessed in an alert, awake and cooperative patient. From the history it is usually obvious whether it is necessary to examine the higher cerebral functions in detail. The ability to give a coherent history suggests normal higher mental function. A patient with sciatica would rightly be dismayed by an examination beginning with asking the patient to name the parts of a watch. However, if the patient is unable to give a coherent history, then cognitive testing is necessary.

General observation
o **Appearance,** e.g. unkempt.
o **Behaviour,** e.g. bewildered, restless, agitated.

o **Emotional state**, e.g. depressed, euphoric, hostile.

Observe, and ask for nurses' and relatives' comments.

Conscious level

If the patient is not fully conscious shake him gently or speak to him loudly.

The Glasgow Coma Scale

The GCS provides a rapid, widely used assessment of level of consciousness. Monitor responses to verbal command or, if no response to painful stimulus, e.g. supraorbital pressure (with thumb nail in supraorbital groove), sternal rub (with knuckles over ribs), nailbed pressure (with thumb nail), twist fold of skin (but do not leave a bruise). It is helpful to record a description of the patient as well as the GCS score.

Add up the total from A, B, C below.

Score

A Eye opening
1 Eyes remain closed
2 Eyes open to pain
3 Eyes open to command
4 Spontaneous with normal blinking

B Verbal response
1 No response
2 Incomprehensible, moaning sounds only
3 Inappropriate—words spoken but no conversation
4 Confused speech
5 Normal speech

C Motor response
1 No response
2 Extensor reflex response to pain—adduction and internal rotation at shoulder, extension at elbows, pronation of forearms
3 Flexor reflex response to pain—withdrawal of limb
4 Localizing: attempts to protect site of pain
5 Voluntary: responds normally to commands

Confusion

If a patient appears confused, move on to assess cognitive state, including disorientation (p. 115). Make sure the patient does not have a receptive aphasia first (see below).

Language/speech

Assess from conversation:

O **Is there difficulty in articulation?**

If necessary, ask patient to say 'British Constitution', 'West Register Street'.

— **Dysarthria**
- — cerebellar — scanning or staccato
- — lower motor neuron
- — palatal palsy — nasal
- — upper motor neuron — slow, 'spastic', seen in pseudobulbar palsy
- — acute alcohol poisoning

O **Is there altered voice tone?**
- — extrapyramidal (monotonous and slow)

— **Dysphonia**
- — cord lesion — hoarse
- — hysterical

O **Is there difficulty in finding the right word?**

— **Dysphasia** or **aphasia** — disorder of use of words as symbols in speech, writing and understanding. Nearly always due to left hemiphere lesion.

N.B. Right- or left-handed? May be right hemisphere lesion if left-handed.

— **Expressive dysphasia** — difficulty finding words; speech slow and hesitant, may use circumlocutions; due to a lesion in Broca's area. Test for by asking patient to name objects you point to, e.g. wrist-watch, pen, tie. Comprehension should be intact.

— **Receptive dysphasia** — speech fluent, but comprehension poor; patient may seem 'confused'. Test for by asking patient to follow commands — a three-step command is a good screening test (e.g. 'please pick up the glass, but first point to the curtain and then the door'). Due to a lesion in Wernicke's area.

- **Mixed dysphasia**—most common; spontaneous speech scanty, small vocabulary, often with wrong words used, comprehension impaired. There are also other dysphasias produced by interruption of the connecting pathways between the speech centres.
- **Mutism**—no speech at all. This may be due to aphasia, anarthria, psychiatric disease or occasionally diffuse cerebral pathology.

Other defects occurring in absence of motor or sensory dysfunction

- **Dyslexia**—inappropriate difficulty with reading. Read few lines from newspaper (having established that comprehension and expressive speech are intact).
- **Dysgraphia**—loss of ability to write.
- **Acalculia**—loss of ability to do mental and written sums.
- **Apraxia**—inability to perform a purposeful task when no motor or sensory loss, e.g. opening matchbox, waving goodbye. Apraxia for dressing is common in *diffuse brain disease*. Inability to draw five-pointed star occurs in *hepatic pre-coma*.
- **Agnosia**—inability to recognize objects (e.g. a key or coin when placed in hand. Tactile agnosia = **astereognosis**).
- **Parietal lobe lesions**—especially right, cause spatial difficulties; getting lost in familiar places, inability to lay table or draw or make patterns with matches, neglect of left side of space, or of half of body.

Cognitive function

Take account of any evidence you have about the patient's intelligence, education and interests.

'Cognitive' is a term that covers **orientation, thought processes and logic. Regular use of a simple mental state test is suggested—examples are shown in Appendix 3.** The section below describes some aspects of cognitive testing in more detail.

Orientation

o **Check awareness of:**
   - **time**: 'What day is it?' (time, month, year)
   - **place**: 'Where are you?'

— **person**: 'What is your name?'

> **Disorientation** suggests *acute organic state* or *dementia. Depressed patients* may be unwilling to reply although they know the answers.

Attention and calculation

O Tests of concentration include asking the patient to take away 7 from 100, 7 from 93, etc.; 20 minus 3 in another simpler version of this test; or by asking for the months of the year backwards, or by spelling the word 'world' backwards.

> **Concentration** may be impaired with many *cerebral abnormalities especially delirium, depression* and *anxiety.*

Memory
Immediate recall—digit span

O Repeat digits spoken slowly. Start with easy short sequence and then increase the numbers. Most people manage seven digits forwards, five backwards.

Short-term memory
O **Ask patient to tell you:**
- what he had for breakfast
- what he did the night before
- what he has read in today's paper
- recent topical news items. This should be geared to the patient's interests, e.g. football results for an avid football fan

> *Demented patients* will be unable to do this. They may **confabulate** (make up impressive stories) to cover their ignorance (particularly likely in alcohol-related dementia).

New memory
O Give a name and address, make sure the patient has learnt it, and then test recall at 5 minutes.

Longer-term memory
O Ask patient:

- for events before illness, e.g. last year, or during last week
- 'What is your address?'

General knowledge
O Assess in relation to anticipated performance from history.
- What is the name of the Queen/President/Prime Minister?
- Name six capital cities.
- What were the dates of the last war?

> In *acute organic states* and *dementia*, new learning, recent memory and reasoning appear to be more impaired than remote memory. Vocabulary is usually well-preserved in *dementia*. In *depression*, patients may be unwilling to reply, and appear demented.

- A history from a relative or employer is very important in early dementia, particularly for ability to function. Demented patients tend not to be able to work appropriately or drive safely; anxious and depressed patients usually can.

Reasoning (abstract thought)
O What would you do if you found a stamped addressed envelope on the ground?

Skull and spine

O **Inspect and palpate skull** if there is any possibility of a head injury.
O **Check neck stiffness** — meningeal irritation (see p. 147)
O **Inspect spine** — usually when examining back of chest.
O If there is any possibility of pathology, stand patient and check all movements of spine.

Cranial nerves

Examine cranial nerves and upper limbs with patient sitting up, preferably on side of bed or on a chair.

I Olfactory

Not normally tested. Occasionally can be useful if there are other neurological defects, including papilloedema, undiagnosed headache or head injury.

> Oil of cloves, peppermint, coffee, etc. — each nostril in turn. It is normal not to be able to name smells, but one smell should be distinguished from another.
>
> Pungent or noxious smells such as ammonia should not be used.
>
> Abnormal:
> - *rhinitis*
> - *head injury*
> - *olfactory groove meningioma*
> - *smoking*

II Optic

Visual acuity
- **Test each eye separately.**
- **Ask patient to read small newspaper print** with each eye separately, **with reading glasses if used.**
- **If sight poor, test formally:**
  - **near vision** — newsprint or **Jaeger type** (each eye in turn) (see Appendix 1).
  - **distant vision — Snellen type** (more precise method) (see Appendix 2).

> Stand patient at 6 m from Snellen's card (each eye in turn). Results expressed as a ratio:
> - 6 — distance of person from card
> - *x* — distance at which patient should be able to read type
>
> i.e. 6/6 is good vision, 6/60 means the smallest type the patient can read is large enough to be normally read at 60 m.
>
> **If the patient cannot read 6/6, try after correction with glasses or pinhole.** Looking through a pinhole in a card obviates refractive errors, analogous to a pinhole camera. If

vision remains poor, suspect a neurological or ophthalmic cause.

A 3 m Snellen chart is shown in Appendix 2.

A pinhole is not effective for correcting near vision for reading.

Visual fields

O Quick method for **temporal peripheral fields** by confrontation of patient and examiner with both eyes open. Always test fields—patients are often unaware of visual loss, the most dramatic of which is Anton's syndrome (blindness with lack of awareness of the blindness).

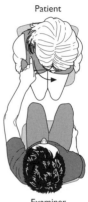

Patient

Examiner

— Sit opposite and ask the patient to look at your nose.

— Examine each eye in turn.

— Bring waggling finger forwards from behind patient's ear in upper and lower lateral quadrants and ask when it can be seen.

   — Normal vision is approximately 100° from axis of eye.

The patient must fully understand the test. The extreme of peripheral vision can be tested with both eyes open, since the nose obstructs vision from the other eye. **If peripheral field appears restricted**, re-test with other eye covered to ensure each eye is being tested separately.

O Quick method for **nasal peripheral fields** by confrontation of patient and examiner with other eye covered.

   — Normal vision is approximately 50° from each axis of eye.

O **Standard method.**

With a small red pinhead held in the plane midway between the patient and examiner. With the other eye covered, compare the visual fields of patient with that of examiner, with pin brought in from temporal or nasal fields.

Defects in the central field can be assessed by the standard method with a small red pin held in the plane midway between the patient and examiner:

— **scotoma**—defects in the central field (*retinal or optic nerve lesion*)

— **enlarged blind spot** (*papilloedema*)

Map by moving pen from inside scotoma or blind spot outwards until red pinhead reappears. This is a crude test and small areas of loss of vision may need to be formally tested with a **perimetry**.

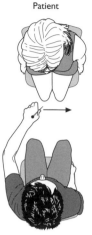

Patient

Examiner

○ **Test for sensory inattention** when fields are full with both eyes open.

— Hold your hands between you and the patient, one opposite each ear and waggle forefingers simultaneously. Ask which moves. With a parietal defect, patient may not recognize movement on one side, although fields are full to formal testing.

○ **In a semiconscious patient a gross homonymous hemianopia** can be detected by a reflex blink to your hand rapidly passing by the eye towards the ear (menace reflex).

— **Homonymous hemianopia** field defect (Fig. 7.1), arising from lesions behind chiasma, is on same side as hemiparesis, if present.

— **Top-quadrant defect**—from *temporal damage* or *occipital lesion*.

— **Lower-quadrant defect**—from *parietal damage* or *occipital lesion*.

— **Bitemporal defect**—from *pituitary lesion*.

Examine the fundi (see p. 35)

○ Lesions particularly relevant to neurological system:

— *optic atrophy*—pale disc and demyelination, e.g. *multiple sclerosis: pressure on nerve*

— *papilloedema*—increased intracranial pressure:

— *tumour*

— *benign intracranial hypertension*

— *hydrocephalus*

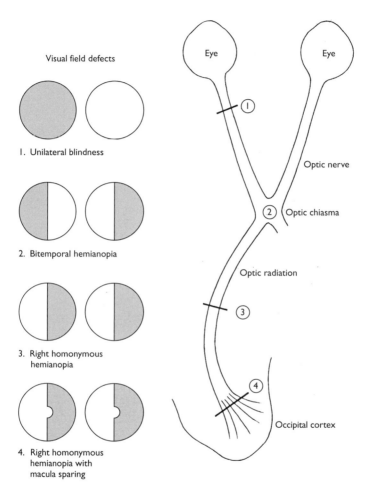

Visual field defects

1. Unilateral blindness

2. Bitemporal hemianopia

3. Right homonymous
   hemianopia

4. Right homonymous
   hemianopia with
   macula sparing

Eye

Eye

Optic nerve

Optic chiasma

Optic radiation

Occipital cortex

Fig. 7.1 Visual field defects.

- *non-communicating* (obstructed outflow via fourth ventricle)
- *communicating*—block of cerebrospinal fluid uptake in spinal cord

O A sensitive test for nystagmus is to ask the patient to cover the other eye during fundoscopy. This removes fixation and can help to elicit nystagmus.

II and III pupils

O **Look at pupils.** Are they round and equal?
   — **Symmetric small pupils:**
   old age
   opiates
   Argyll Robertson pupils (syphilis) are small, irregular, eccentric pupils, reacting to convergence but not light
   pilocarpine eye drops for narrow-angle glaucoma
   iritis
   — **Symmetric large pupils:**
   youth
   alcohol
   sympathomimetics, anxiety
   atropine-like substances
   — **Asymmetric pupils:**
   third-nerve palsy—affected pupil dilated, often with ptosis and diplopia
   Horner's syndrome (sympathetic defect)—affected pupil constricted, often with partial ptosis, enophthalmos and anhydrosis
   iris trauma
   drugs (see above)

O **Light reflex.** Shine bright light from torch into each pupil in turn in a dimly lit room. Do pupils contract equally?
   — *Holmes–Adie pupil*: large, slowly reacting to light.
   — *Afferent defect, ocular or optic nerve blindness*: neither pupil responds to light in blind eye; both respond to light in normal eye.
   — Relative afferent defect
      — direct response appears normal but when light moves from normal to deficient eye, paradoxical dilation of pupil occurs
   — *Efferent defect*—*third-nerve lesion*, pupil does not respond to light in either eye.

O **Accommodation reflex.** Ask patient to look at distant object, and then at your finger 10–15 cm from nose—do pupils contract?

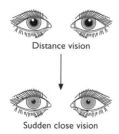

Distance vision

Sudden close vision

— Response to accommodation but not light:
    Argyll Robertson
    Holmes–Adie
    occular blindness
    midbrain lesion
    some recovering *third-nerve lesions*

III Oculomotor

IV Trochlear

VI Abducens

External ocular movements

o **Test the eye movements in the four cardinal directions** (left, right, up, down) and convergence using your finger at 1 m distance. Look for abnormal eye movements.

o **Ask: 'Tell me if you see double'.**

> Upward gaze and convergence are often reduced in unco-operative patients.

o To detect minor lesions:

- **Find direction of gaze with maximum separation of images.**

- **Cover one eye and ask which image has gone.**

> Peripheral image is seen by the eye that is not moving fully. **Peripheral image is displaced in direction of action of weak muscle**, e.g. maximum diplopia on gaze to left. Left eye

sees peripheral image which is displaced laterally. Therefore left lateral rectus is weak.

Looking left

Normal

Left lateral rectus palsy (VI nerve)

Looking ahead

Normal

Left III nerve palsy

- **Diplopia** may be due to a single muscle or nerve lesion (N.B. monocular diplopia usually implies ocular pathology):
  - paralytic strabismus (squint)
    - **III palsy**: ptosis, large fixed pupil, eye can be abducted only; eye is often 'down and out'
    - **IV palsy**: diplopia when eye looks down or inwards
    - **VI palsy**: abduction paralysed, diplopia when looking to side of lesion
  - **concomitant non-paralytic strabismus**, e.g. *childhood ocular lesion* — constant angle between eyes. Usually no double vision as one eye ignored (amblyopic)

Looking right

Looking ahead

Normal

Concomitant strabismus with amblyopic left eye

- **conjugate ocular palsy**
    - *supranuclear palsies* affecting coordination rather than muscle weakness. Inability to look in particular direction, usually upwards
    - *intranuclear lesion*: convergence normal but cannot adduct eyes on lateral gaze

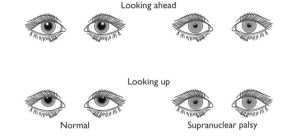

Looking ahead

Looking up

Normal   Supranuclear palsy

- if patient sees double in all directions
    - may be *third-nerve palsy*
    - *thyroid muscle disease* — worse in morning
    - myasthenia gravis — worse in evening
    - manifest strabismus

Ptosis

Drooping of upper eyelid can be:
- complete — *third-nerve palsy*
- incomplete
    - *partial third-nerve palsy*
    - muscular weakness, e.g. *myasthenia gravis* (from anti-acetylcholine receptor antibodies)
    - sympathetic tone decreased — *Horner's syndrome* (also small pupils — enophthalmos and decreased sweating on face)
    - partial Horner's syndrome (small irregular pupils with ptosis) in *autonomic neuropathy of diabetes and syphilis*
    - lid swelling
    - levator dysinsertion syndrome (from chronic contact lens use)

Nystagmus

This is an unsteady eye movement. The flickering movement is labelled by the direction of fast movement.

○ **Test first in the neutral position and then with the eyes deviated to right, left and upwards.** Keep object within binocular field as nystagmus is often normal in extremes of gaze.

Characterized as primary when present with eyes at rest, or as gaze evoked, i.e. when produced by eye movement. Nystagmus is easier to detect with fixation removed. This can be done at bedside during ophthalmoscopy (see above). Remember, the nystagmus will appear in the opposite direction.

- – Cerebellar nystagmus
  - – fast movement to side of gaze (on both sides)
  - – increased when looking to lesion
    - – *cerebellar or brainstem lesion or drugs (ethanol, phenytoin)*

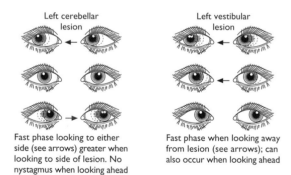

Left cerebellar lesion

Left vestibular lesion

Fast phase looking to either side (see arrows) greater when looking to side of lesion. No nystagmus when looking ahead

Fast phase when looking away from lesion (see arrows); can also occur when looking ahead

- – Vestibular nystagmus
  - – fast movement only in one direction — away from lesion
  - – reduced by fixation if peripheral in origin
  - – more marked when looking away from lesion
    - – *inner ear, vestibular disease or brainstem lesion*
  - – labyrinthine nystagmus may be positional — particularly in benign positional vertigo, and can be induced by hyperextension and rotation of the neck (Hallpike manoeuvre) which after a

latency of a few seconds will produce a vertical/torsional type of nystagmus for about 10–15 seconds, along with symptoms of vertigo

— **Congenital nystagmus** — constant horizontal wobbling.
— Downbeat nystagmus — foramen magnum lesion or Wernicke's disease.
— Retraction nystagmus — midbrain lesion.
— Complex nystagmus — brainstem disease, usually multiple sclerosis.

Saccades

This is the rapid eye movement used to change eye position. It is tested in the horizontal and vertical planes, by asking the patient to switch fixation between two targets (e.g. the examiner's fingers). Slow saccades may be seen in a variety of disorders including degenerative disorders such as progressive supranuclear palsy.

V Trigeminal

Sensory V

o **Test light touch in all three divisions.** A light touch with one's fingers is often adequate. Pinprick usually only if needed to delineate anaesthetic area.

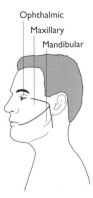

Ophthalmic
Maxillary
Mandibular

Corneal reflex—sensory V and motor VII

O **Ask the patient to look up and touch the cornea with a wisp of cotton wool.** Both eyes should blink. Remember the cornea is clear; do not test the sclera!

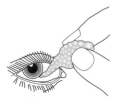

The corneal reflex is easily prompted incorrectly by eliciting the 'eyelash' or 'menace' reflex.

Motor V—muscles of jaw

O **Ask the patient to open his mouth against resistance,** and look to see if jaw descends in midline. Palsy of the nerve causes deviation of the jaw to the side of the lesion.

Fifth-nerve palsies are very rare in isolation.

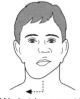

Weak right pterygoid

O **Jaw jerk**—only if other neurological findings, e.g. upper motor neuron lesion. Increased jaw jerk is only present if there is a bilateral upper motor neuron fifth-nerve lesion, e.g. *bilateral strokes* or *pseudobulbar palsy*.

Put your forefinger gently on the patient's loosely opened jaw. Tap

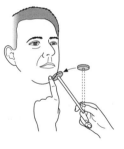

your finger gently with a tendon hammer. Explain the test to the patient or relaxation of his jaw will be impossible. A brisk jerk is a positive finding.

VII Facial

O **Ask the patient to:**
- raise his eyebrows
- close his eyes tightly
- show you his teeth

Demonstrate these to the patient yourself if necessary.

> **Lower motor neuron lesion**: all muscles on the side of the lesion are affected, e.g. *Bell's palsy*: widened palpebral fissure, weak blink, drooped mouth.

> **Upper motor neuron lesion**: only the lower muscles are affected, i.e. mouth drops to one side but eyebrows raise normally. This is because the part of the facial nucleus controlling the upper half of the face is bilaterally innervated. This abnormality is very common in a hemiparesis.

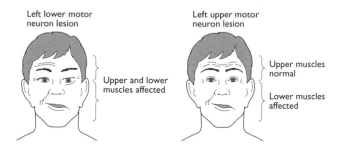

Left lower motor neuron lesion — Upper and lower muscles affected

Left upper motor neuron lesion — Upper muscles normal / Lower muscles affected

O **Taste** (chorda tympani): can only be tested easily on anterior two-thirds of the tongue.

VIII Auditory

Vestibular

No easy bedside test for this nerve except looking for nystagmus.

Acoustic

o **Block one ear by pressing the tragus. Whisper numbers increasingly loudly until the patient can repeat them. A ticking watch may be more useful.**

> **Rinne's test.** Place a high-pitched vibrating tuning fork on the mastoid (I in figure). When the patient says the sound stops, hold the fork at the meatus (2 in figure).
>
> — If still heard: air conduction > bone conduction (normal or nerve deafness).
>
> — If not heard: air conduction < bone conduction (middle-ear conduction defect).

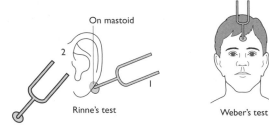

On mastoid

Rinne's test

Weber's test

> **Weber's test.** Hold a vibrating tuning fork in the middle of the patient's forehead. If the sound is heard to one side, middle-ear deafness exists on that side or the opposing ear has nerve deafness.

IX Glossopharyngeal

o **Ask patient to say 'Ahh'** and watch for symmetrical upwards movement of uvula—pulled away from weak side.

o **Touch the back of the pharynx with an orange-stick** or spatula gently. If the patient gags the nerve is intact.

> This gag reflex depends on the IX and X nerve, the former being the sensory side and the latter the

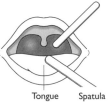

Tongue   Spatula

motor aspect. It is frequently absent with ageing and abuse of tobacco.

X Vagus

○ **Ask if the patient can swallow normally.**

There are so many branches of the vagus nerve that it is impossible to be sure it is all functioning normally. If the vagus is seriously damaged, swallowing is a problem; spillage into the lungs may occur. Swallowing can be assessed by asking the patient to take a small drink of water. Observe the patient. Coughing on attempted swallow indicates a high risk of aspiration. Check speech afterwards—a change of voice quality ('wet' speech) indicates pooling of fluids on the vocal cords, and again indicates a high risk of aspiration. Check a voluntary cough—this can become quiet and ineffective.

○ Check dysarthria (see p. 114).

XI Accessory

○ **Ask the patient to flex neck,** pressing his chin against your resisting hand. Observe if both sternomastoids contract normally.

○ **Ask the patient to raise both shoulders.** If he cannot, the trapezius muscle is not functioning.

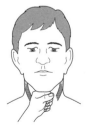 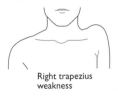

Right trapezius weakness

Failure of the trapezius on one side is often associated with a *hemiplegia* (*particulary anterior cerebral artery infarctions*). Traumatic cutting of the accessory nerve used to occur when tuberculous lymph glands of the neck were being excised.

o **Ask the patient to turn the head against your resisting hand.**
This tests the contralateral sternomastoid, and can help to demonstrate normal motor functioning in a hysterical hemiplegia.

XII Hypoglossal

o **Ask the patient to put out his tongue.** If it
protrudes to one side, this is the side of the
weakness, e.g. deviating to left on protrusion
from left hypoglossal lesion.

o **Look for fasciculation or wasting** with
mouth open.

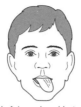

Left hypoglossal lesion

Limbs and trunk: motor, tone, coordination and reflexes

General inspection

o **Look at the patient's resting and standing posture:**
— *hemiplegia*—flexed upper limb, extended lower limb
— *wrist drop*—radial nerve palsy
o **Look for abnormal movements:**
— tremor
— *Parkinson's*—coarse rhythmical tremor at rest, lessens on
movement
— essential tremor—tremor present on action; look at outstretched hands
— *chorea*—abrupt, involuntary repetitive semi-purposeful
movement
— *athetosis*—slow, continuous writhing movement of limb
o **Look for muscle wasting.** Check distribution:
— symmetrical, e.g. *Duchenne muscular dystrophy*
— asymmetrical, e.g. *poliomyelitis*
— proximal, e.g. *limb-girdle muscular dystrophy*
— distal, e.g. *peripheral neuropathy*
— generalized, e.g. *motor neuron disease*
— localized, e.g. with *joint disease*

○ **Look for fasciculation.** This is irregular involuntary contractions of small bundles of muscle fibres.

> This is typical of denervation, e.g. *motor neuron disease when it is widespread*. It is caused by the death of anterior horn cells.

○ **Ask the patient to hold both his arms straight out in front with the palms up and eyes shut.** Observe gross weakness, posture and whether arms remain stationary:
  — *hypotonic posture* — wrist flexed and fingers extended
  — *drift* — gradually upwards with sensory loss, especially parietal lobe
  — gradually downwards with pronation indicates *pyramidal weakness*
  — downward without pronation can be seen in hysteria or in profound proximal muscle weakness
  — athetoid tremors — sensory loss (peripheral nerve) or cerebellar disease

○ **Tap both arms downwards.** They should reflexly return to their former position.

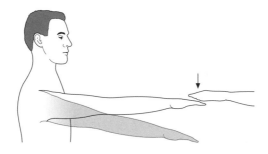

> If the arm overswings in its return to its position, *weakness* or *cerebellar dysfunction* may be present.

○ **Ask the patient to do fast finger movements**: 'Play a quick tune on the piano', demonstrating this yourself. Clumsy movements can be a sensitive index of a slight *pyramidal lesion*. The dominant side should always be quicker than the non-dominant.

Tone

Always check tone before you assess strength. This is a difficult test to perform as patients often do not relax. Try to distract the patient with conversation.

O **Ask the patient to relax his arm and then you flex and extend his wrist or elbow.** Move through a wide arc moderately slowly, at irregular intervals to prevent patient cooperation.

O **Ask the patient to let the limb go loose, lift it up and move at knee joint** (hip and ankle if required).

> Difficult to assess in the legs because patients often cannot relax. Ankle clonus can be assessed at same time (see below).

Hypertonia (increased tone):

- **pyramidal**: more obvious in flexion of upper limbs and extension of lower limbs. Occasionally 'clasp knife', i.e. diminution of tone during movement
- **extrapyramidal**: uniform 'lead pipe' rigidity. If associated with tremor the movement feels like a 'cog wheel'
- **hysterical**: increases with increased movement

Hypotonia (decreased tone):

lower motor neuron lesion

recent *upper motor neuron lesion*

cerebellar lesion

unconsciousness

Muscle power

O **For screening purposes, examine two distal muscles, one flexor and one extensor (e.g. finger flexion and extension), and two proximal muscles in each limb. Compare each side.** Confirm the weakness suspected by palpation of the muscle.

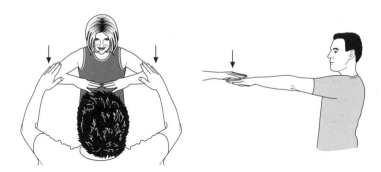

○ If patient is in bed, start examination by asking him to:
   — raise both arms
   — raise one leg off the bed
   — raise the other leg off the bed
○ Test power at joints against your own strength—shoulder, elbow, wrist.

> Power at main joints cannot normally be overcome by permissible force.

○ **If there is weakness or other neurological signs in a limb, test individual muscle groups:**
   — shoulder—abduction, extension, flexion
   — elbow—flexion, extension
   — wrist—flexion, extension: 'Hold wrists up, don't let me push them down'
   — finger—flexion, grasp, extension, adduction (put a piece of paper between straight fingers held in extension and ask the patient to hold it, as you remove it), abduction (with fingers in extension, ask patient to spread them apart against your force).
   — hip—flexion (ask patient to lift leg, 'don't let me push down') and extension (ask patient to keep leg straight on bed, and try to lift at ankle); occasionally also abduction and adduction

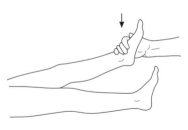

- knee—flexion, extension
- ankle—plantarflexion, dorsiflexion, eversion, inversion

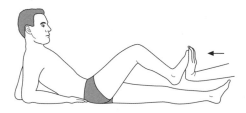

Only severe weakness will be detected because legs are stronger than arms. If no weakness is detected and patient is complaining of weakness, then more sensitive tests can be helpful, e.g. walking on tiptoes, heels, arising from a squat position, hopping on either leg.

Occasionally patients will have hysterical weakness. A useful test is Hoover's sign. This is tested by placing your hand under the ankle of the patient's paralysed leg. The patient is first asked to extend the paralysed leg (which should produce no effort), and then by asking for hip flexion of the non-paralysed leg, resulting in contraction of the 'paralysed' hip extensor (a reflex fixation that we all do). Unlike other tests for non-organic illness, this test demonstrates normalcy in the paralysed limb.

Strength is usually graded as follows:

0 No active contraction.
1 Visible as palpable contraction with no active movement.
2 Movement with gravity eliminated, i.e. in horizontal direction.
3 Movement against gravity.
4 Movement against gravity plus resistance: it may be subdivided into 4– to 4+.
5 Normal power.

○ Look for patterns of weakness:
- *hemiplegia*—muscles weak all down one side
- *monoplegia*—weakness of one limb
- *paraplegia*—weakness of both lower limbs

- *tetraplegia*—weakness of all four limbs
- *myasthenia*—weakness developing after repeated contractions—most obvious in smaller muscles, e.g. repeated blinking (see ptosis. p. 125)
- proximal muscles, e.g. myopathy
- nerve root distribution, e.g. disc prolapse
- nerve distribution, e.g. wrist drop from radial nerve palsy

Coordination

O **Ask the patient to touch his nose with his index finger.**

O **With the patient's eyes open, ask him to touch his nose, then your finger which is held up in front of him.** This can be repeated rapidly with your finger moving from place to place in front of him.

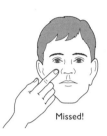

Missed!

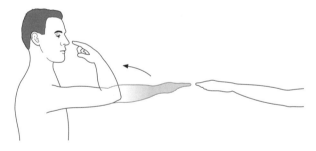

Past pointing and marked intention tremor in the absence of muscular weakness suggests *cerebellar dysfunction*. If you suspect a cerebellar abnormality check rapid alternating movements (*dysdiadochokinesia*):

- **fast rotation of the hands** (supination and pronation)
- **tapping back of other hand as quickly as possible**

O Ask the patient to run the heel of one leg up and down the shin of the other leg. Lack of coordination will be apparent.

O Gait may become broad based, and patient unable to perform a tandem gait (heel–toe walking).

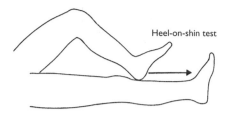

Heel-on-shin test

Tendon reflexes

O Place arms comfortably by side with elbows flexed and hand on upper abdomen. Tell the patient to relax.

O **Supinator reflex:** tap the distal end of the radius with a tendon hammer.

O **Biceps reflex:** tap your forefinger or thumb over biceps tendon.

O **Triceps reflex:** hold arm across chest to tap the triceps tendon.

O **Knee reflexes:** by passing left forearm behind both knees, supporting them partly flexed. Ask the patient to let leg go loose and tap the tendons below patella.

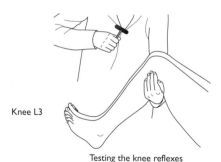

Knee L3

Testing the knee reflexes

O **Ankle reflex:** by flexing the knee and abducting the leg. Apply gentle pressure to the ball of the foot, with it at a right angle and tap the tendon.

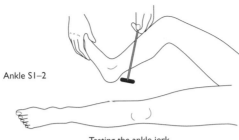

Ankle S1–2

Testing the ankle jerk

Ankle jerks are often absent in the elderly.

o **Compare sides** (right versus left; arms versus legs).

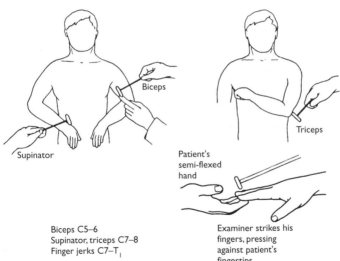

Biceps

Triceps

Supinator

Patient's
semi-flexed
hand

Biceps C5–6
Supinator, triceps C7–8
Finger jerks C7–T₁

Examiner strikes his
fingers, pressing
against patient's
fingertips

It is essential for the patient to relax and this is not always easy,
particularly in the elderly.

Increased jerks—*upper motor neuron lesion* (e.g.
hemiparesis).

Decreased jerks—*lower motor neuron lesion* or *acute upper
motor neuron lesion.*

Clonus—pressure stretching a muscle group causes rhythmical involuntary contraction. If a brisk reflex is obtained, test for clonus. A sharp, then sustained dorsiflexion of the foot by pressure on ball of foot may result in the foot 'beating' for many seconds. Clonus confirms an increased tendon jerk and suggests an *upper motor neuron lesion*. A few symmetrical beats may be normal.

Plantar reflexes

○ **Tell patient what you are doing, and scratch the side of the sole with a noxious but not injurious implement.** An orange stick is quite useful. Watch for flexion or extension of the toes.

Normal plantar responses—flexion of all toes.

Extensor (Babinski) response—slow extension of the big toe with spreading of the other toes. Withdrawal from pain or tickle is rapid and not abnormal. In individuals with sensitive feet, the reflex can be elicited by noxious stimuli elsewhere in the leg; stroking the lateral aspect of the foot can be very useful, or testing pinprick sensation on the dorsum of the great toe.

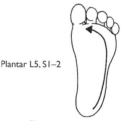

Plantar L5, S1–2

Plantar response stimulus

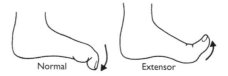

Normal   Extensor

Trunk

○ **The superficial abdominal reflexes rarely need to be tested.**

– Lightly stroke each quadrant with an orange-stick or the back of your fingernail. These reflexes are absent or decreased in an upper or lower motor neuron lesion. They are typically absent in multiple sclerosis.

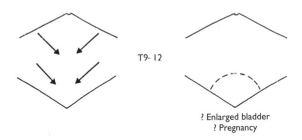

T9- 12

? Enlarged bladder
? Pregnancy

o **Cremasteric reflex T12–L1.**
  — Stroke inside of leg—induces testis to rise from cremaster muscle contraction.
o **Palpate the bladder.**
  The patient with a distended bladder will feel very uncomfortable as you palpate it.

  Many neurological lesions, sensory or motor, will lead to a distended bladder, giving the patient *retention with overflow incontinence.*
o Examine the strength of the abdominal muscles by asking the patient to attempt to sit up without using his hands.

Sensation
If there are no grounds to expect sensory loss, sensation can be rapidly examined.

  Briefly examine each extremity. Success depends on making the patient understand what you are doing. Children are the best sensory witnesses and dons the worst. The examination is very subjective. As in the motor examination, one is looking for patterns of loss, e.g. nerve root (dermatome), nerve, sensory level (spinal cord), glove/stocking (peripheral neuropathy), dissociation (i.e. pain and temperature versus vibration and proprioception—e.g. syringomyelia).

Vibration sense

o **Test vibration sense** using a 128/s tuning fork. Place the fork on the sternum first so that the patient appreciates what vibration is. Then place the tuning fork on the distally on each extremity. The patient should feel the sensation as long as the examiner (assuming the examiner is normal!). The occasional patient will claim to feel vibration when it is absent—if this is suspected, try a non-vibrating tuning fork; if they feel it vibrate, testing is not valid. Vibration often diminishes with age, probably as part of age-related neuropathy.

Position sense—proprioception

o Show patient what you are doing. 'I am going to move your finger/toe up or down' [doing so]. I want you to tell me up or down each time I move it. Now close your eyes'.

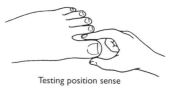

Testing position sense

o Hold distal to joint, and side to side, with your forefinger and thumb, and make small movements in an irregular, not alternate, sequence, e.g. up, up, down, down, up, down.

Normal threshold is very low—the smallest, slowest passive movement you can produce in the terminal phalanges should always be correctly detected.

Pain

o Take a clean or sterile pin and do not re-use same pin on another patient.

o Touch the sharp end on the skin. Do not draw blood. Patient's eyes can be open.

o 'Does this feel sharp, like a pinprick?'

If you find sensory loss, map out that area by proceeding from abnormal to normal area of skin.

If you are uncertain about sensory loss, another (cumbersome) method is to ask the patient to close his eyes, and put either the blunt or sharp end of the pin on the skin in an irregular pattern and ask which is which.

Light touch

o Close patient's eyes.
o 'Say "yes" when I touch you with tactile filaments, 1 g, 10 g and 75 g pressure, or a wisp of cotton wool.' Touch at irregular intervals. Compare sides of body.

> **Thermal sensation** is not examined routinely. Tests with hot and cold water in glass tubes cannot be standardized. Find an area where hot is called cold or vice versa and draw tube along skin until true temperature is recognized.
>
> **Two-point discrimination.** Normal threshold on fingertip is 2 mm. If sensory impairment is peripheral or in cord, a raised threshold is found, e.g. 5 mm. If cortical, no threshold is found.
>
> **Stereognosis** tested by placing coins, keys, pen top, etc. in hand and, with eyes closed, patient attempts to identify by feeling.
>
> **Sensory inattention** is best found with pin, not touch. Bilateral simultaneous symmetrical pinpricks are felt only on the normal side, while each is felt if applied separately. Found in cortical lesions.

Dermatomes

Most are easily detected with pin. Map out from area of impaired sensation.

Note in arms: **middle finger—C7** and dermatomes either side symmetrical up to mid upper arm.

Note in legs: **lateral border of foot and heel (S1)**, back of legs and anal region have sacral supply.

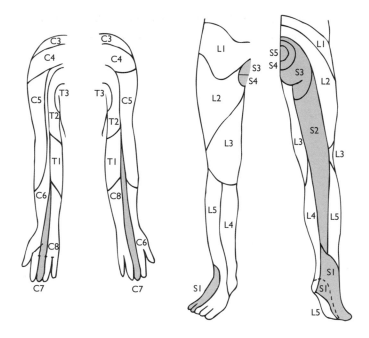

Gait (see p. 45)

o **Observe the patient as he walks in. If ataxia is suspected but not seen on ordinary walking, ask the patient to do heel-to-toe walking. (Demonstrate it yourself.)**

There are many examples of abnormal gait.

Parkinson's disease. Stooped posture with most joints flexed, with small shuffling steps without swinging arms; tremor of hands.

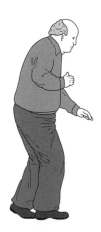

Spastic gait. Scraping toe on one or both sides as patient walks, moving foot in lateral arc to prevent this.

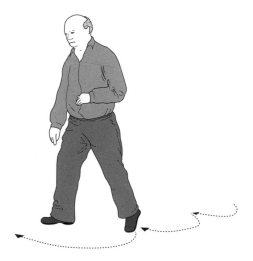

Sensory ataxia. High stepping gait, with slapping-down of feet. Seen with peripheral neuropathy.

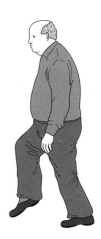

Cerebellar gait. Feet wide apart as patient walks.

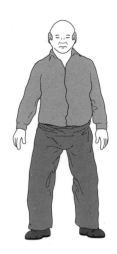

Foot drop. Toe scrapes on ground in spite of excessive lifting-up of leg on affected side.

Shuffling gait. Multiple little steps—typical of diffuse cerebral vascular disease.

Hysterical gait. Usually wild lurching without falling.

Romberg's test is often performed at this time but is mainly a test of position sense. Ask the patient to stand upright with his feet together and close his eyes. If there is any falling noted, the test is positive.

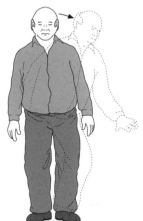

Elderly patients may fail this test and *hysterics* may fall sideways but stop just before they topple over. Test positive with posterior column loss of *tabes dorsalis of syphilis*. Anxious patients may sway excessively; try distracting by testing stereognosis at the same time — the excess swaying may disappear!

Background information

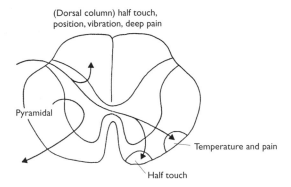

(Dorsal column) half touch, position, vibration, deep pain

Pyramidal

Temperature and pain

Half touch

Dorsal column loss of sensation
- Decreased position, vibration and deep pain sensation (squeeze Achilles' tendon).
- Touch often not lost, as half carried in anterior column.

Cortical loss of sensation
Defect shown by deficient:
- position sense
- tactile discrimination
- sensory inattention

Signs of meningeal irritation
- Neck rigidity — try to flex neck. Resistance or pain?
- Kernig's sign — not as sensitive as neck rigidity.

Pain in back

Straight-leg-raising for sciatica

— Lift straight leg until pain in back. Then slightly lower until no pain and then dorsiflex foot to 'stretch' sciatic nerve until there is pain.

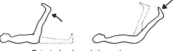

Pain in back and down leg

Summary of common illnesses

Lower motor neuron lesion

— wasting
— fasciculation
— hypotonia
— power diminished
— absent reflexes
— ± sensory loss
— **T1 palsy**—weakness of intrinsic muscles of hand: finger abduction and adduction, thumb abduction (cf. median nerve palsy and ulnar nerve palsy)
  — sensory loss: medial forearm
— **median nerve palsy**—abductor pollicis brevis weakness (other thenar muscles may be weak)
  — sensory loss: thumb, first two fingers, palmar surface
— **ulnar nerve palsy**—interversion, hypothenar muscles wasted, weakness of finger abduction and adduction; claw-hand, cannot extend fingers

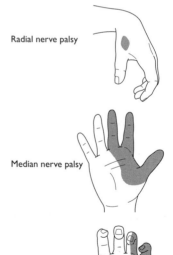

Radial nerve palsy

Median nerve palsy

Ulnar nerve palsy

- sensory loss: half fourth, all fifth fingers palmar surface
- **radial nerve palsy** — wrist drop
    - sensory loss: small area/dorsal web of thumb
- **L5 palsy** — foot drop and weak inversion; sensory loss on medial aspect of foot
- **peroneal nerve palsy** — foot drop and weak eversion; minor sensory loss of dorsum of foot
- **S1 palsy** — cannot stand on toes, sensory loss of lateral aspect of foot, absent ankle reflex

Upper motor neuron lesion

- no wasting
- extended arms — hand drifts down
- overswing when hands are tapped
- rapid alternating movements performed slowly: clumsy 'piano playing'
- hypertonia
    - spastic flexion of upper limbs, extension of lower limbs
    - clasp knife
- power diminished
- increased tendon reflexes ($\pm$ clonus)
- extensor plantar response
- $\pm$ sphincter disturbance
- spastic gait
    - extended stiff leg with foot drop
    - arm does not swing, held flexed

N.B. Check 'level' first, then pathology.

Cerebellar dysfunction

- no wasting
- hypotonia with overswing; irregularity of movements
- intention tremor
- inability to execute rapid alternating movements smoothly (dysdiadochokinesia)
- ataxic gait

- nystagmus
- scanning or staccato speech
- incoordination not improved by sight (whereas is with sensory defect)

Extrapyramidal dysfunction — Parkinson's disease

Bradykinesia, rigidity, tremor and postural instability are the cardinal features:

- flexed posture of body, neck, arms and legs
- expressionless, impassive facies, staring eyes
- 'pill-rolling' tremor of hands at rest
- delay in initiating movements
- tone — 'lead pipe' rigidity, possibly with 'cog-wheeling'
- normal power and sensation
- speech quiet and monotonal
- gait — shuffling small steps, possibly with difficulty starting or stopping
- postural instability: test by having patient standing comfortably. Stand behind the patient and give a sharp tug backwards. Normal patients should show a slight sway; taking steps backwards, particularly multiple steps, is abnormal

Multiple sclerosis

- **evidence of 'different lesions in space and time' from history and examination. Usually affects cerebral white matter.** Common sites:
  - optic atrophy — optic neuritis
  - nystagmus — vestibular or cerebellar tracts
  - brisk jaw jerk — pyramidal lesion above fifth nerve
- cerebellar signs in arms or gait — cerebellar tracts
- upper motor neuron signs in arms or legs — pyramidal, right or left (absent superficial abdominal reflexes)
- transverse myelitis with sensory level — indicates level of lesion
- urine retention — usually sensory tract
- sensory perception loss — sensory tract

System-oriented examination

'Examine the higher cerebral functions'

- general appearance
- consciousness level
- mood
- speech
- cognitive
  - confusion
  - orientation
  - attention/calculation
  - memory—short-term, long-term
  - reasoning—understanding of proverb

'Examine the cranial nerves'

I	smell (only test if the hint of smell bottles are present)
II	visual acuity
	visual fields
	fundi
III, IV, VI	ptosis
	nystagmus
	eye movements
	pupils
V	sensory face
	corneal reflex
	jaw muscles/jerk
VII	face muscles—upper/lower motor neuron defect (taste if taste bottles are provided)
VIII	hearing
	Rinne/Weber tests
	nystagmus
IX, X	palate
	swallowing
	(taste—posterior third of tongue)
XI	trapezius
XII	tongue wasting

'Examine the arms neurologically'

- O *inspect*:
    - abnormal position
    - wasting
    - fasciculation
    - tremor/athetosis
- O ask patient to extend arms in front, palms up, keep them there with eyes closed, then check:
    - posture/drift
    - tap back of wrists to assess whether position is stable
    - fast finger movements (pyramidal)
    - touch nose (coordination) — finger–nose test
    - 'Hold my fingers. Pull me up. Push me away'
- O tone
- O muscle power — each group if indicated
- O reflexes
- O sensation
    - light touch
    - pinprick
    - vibration
    - proprioception

'Examine the legs neurologically'

- O *inspect*:
    - abnormal positions
    - wasting
    - fasciculation
- O 'Lift one leg off the bed'
- O 'Lift other leg off the bed'
- O coordination — heel–toe
- O tone
- O power — 'Pull up toes. Push down toes'
- O reflexes
- O plantar reflexes
- O sensation (as hands)

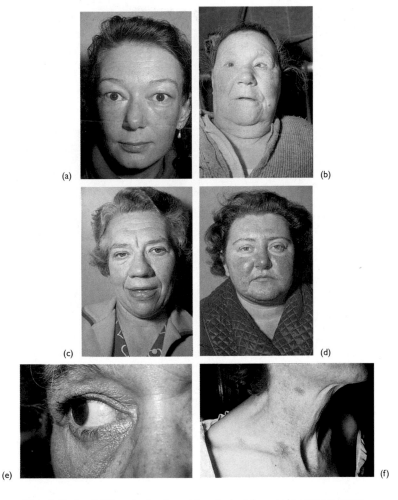

Plate 1: Facies (a) Thyrotoxicosis—wide palpebral fissures in a tense person. (b) Myxoedema—puffy face, thin dry hair and dry skin in a sluggish person. (c) Acromegaly—coarse features with thick lips, enlarged nose and thickened skin. (d) Cushing's syndrome—plethoric, round face. (e) Jaundice—yellow sclerae. (f) Spider naevi in cirrhosis—talangiectasia radiating from central arteriole.

[facing page 152]

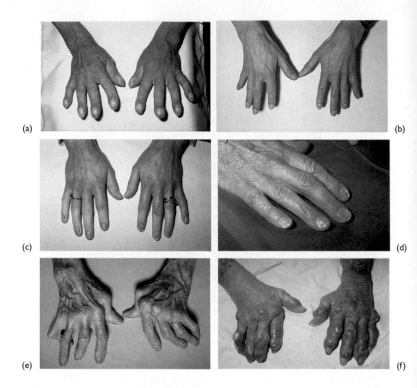

Plate 2: Hands (a) Finger clubbing—gross with carcinoma of bronchus. (b) Congenital cyanotic heart disease—dusky, cyanotic hands with mild clubbing. (c) Raynaud's syndrome—white/blue fingers induced by cold. (d) Koilonychia from iron deficiency—spoon-shaped nails. (e) Rheumatoid arthritis—symmetrically enlarged metacarpophalangeal and interphalangeal joints, with secondary wasting of interossei muscles and subluxation of fingers from snapped dorsal tendons. (f) Gout—asymmetrical swelling of joints with subcutaneous 'tophi' of uric acid deposits.

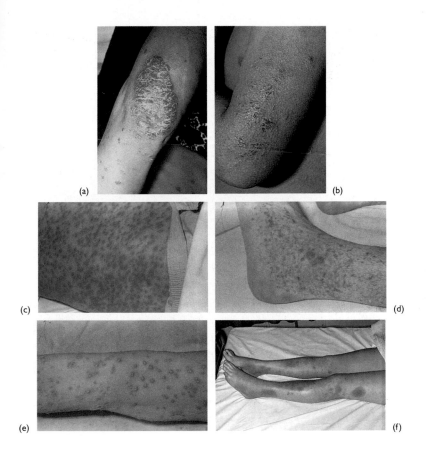

Plate 3: Skin (a) Psoriasis—circumscribed plaque with scales. (b) Eczema on upper arm—diffuse erythema and scratch marks, with small blisters and fine scales that cannot be seen on this photo. (c) Ampicillin rash—patchy red macules that blanche on pressure. (d) Henoch–Schönlein syndrome—macular/papular rash including petechiae that do not blanche on pressure. (e) Chicken pox—peripheral circumscribed, erythematous papules with central blister. (f) Erythema nodosum—approximately 5–10 cm across swellings in dermis of shins with red, warm surfaces.

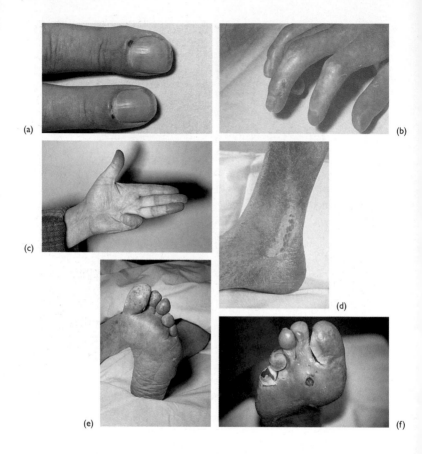

Plate 4: Extremities (a) Nail-fold infarcts from polyarteritis—small black areas, often associated with splinter haemorrhages in nails. (b) Scleroderma—thick shiny skin and limiting joint movements with ulcers from subcutaneous calcification. (c) Dupuytren's contraction—thickened palmar skin attached to the tendons. (d) Healing varicose ulcer—classic site in lower leg medially with pigmentation from venous stasis. (e) Ischaemic toes from acute arterial insufficiency—white toes becoming blue, with erythematous reaction at demarcation. (f) Diabetic foot—shiny, dry skin with ulcer from abnormal pressure point from motor neuropathy and painless, unsuspected blister on toe.

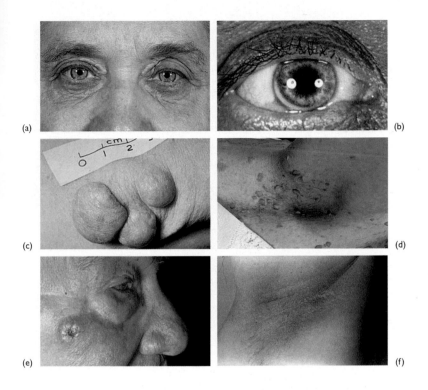

(a)

(b)

(c)

(d)

(e)

(f)

Plate 5: Dyslipidaemia and skin lesions (a) Xanthelasma–cholesterol deposits—suggests raised lipids in younger persons, but lipids are often normal in the elderly. (b) Corneal arcus—same age relationship as xanthelasma. (c) Tuberous xanthoma of elbows in homozygous familial hypercholesterolaemia—also occur in tendons and it signifies very high cholesterol levels. (d) Neurofibromatosis Type 1 (von Recklinghausen's disease)—multiple cutaneous fibroma. (e) Rodent ulcer—raised, shiny papule with telangiectasia on the surface with a central ulcer. (f) Acanthosis nigricans in the armpit—thickened epidermis from gross insulin resistance which also occurs on the neck.

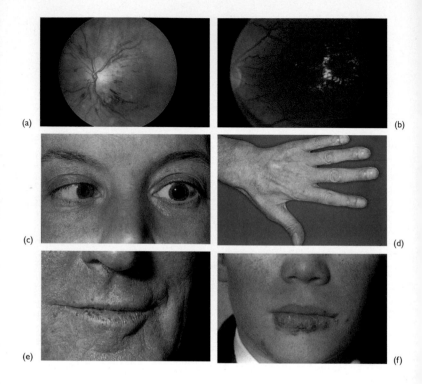

Plate 6: Retinae, palsies, lips (a) Hypertensive retinopathy—narrow arteries, flame haemorrhages and an early papilloedema with an indistinct disc margin. (b) Diabetic retinopathy—hard exudates in a ring (circinate). (c) Left sixth nerve lesion—the patient is looking to the left, but there is no lateral movement of the left eye. (d) Wasted interossei and hypothenar eminence from an ulna nerve or T_1 lesion. (e) Osler–Weber–Rendu syndrome—telangiectasia on the lip in a patient with haematemasis. (f) Herpes simplex on lips ('cold sores')—these can erupt with other illnesses.

O Romberg test
O gait and tandem gait

'Examine the arms or legs'

O *inspect*:
- colour
- skin/nail changes
- ulcers
- wasting (are both arms and legs involved?)
- joints
O palpate:
- temperature, pulses
- lumps (see above)
- joints
  - active movements
  - feel for crepitus, e.g. hand over knee during flexion
  - passive movements (do not hurt patient)
- reflexes
- sensation

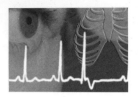

CHAPTER 8

Assessment of Disability Including Care of the Elderly

Introduction

It is important, particularly in the elderly, to **assess whether the patient has a disability**:

- which interferes with normal life and aspirations
- which makes the patient dependent on others
    - requires temporary assistance for specific problems
    - occasional or regular assistance long-term
    - supervised accommodation
    - nursing home with 24-hour care

It is necessary to assess the following in a patient:

o **ability to do day-to-day functions**
o **mental ability, including confusion or dementia**
o **emotional state and drive**

The descriptive terms used for disability have specific definitions in a World Health Organization classification.

- **Impairment**—any loss or abnormality of anatomical, physiological or psychological function, i.e. **systems or parts of body that do not work.**
- **Disability**—any restrictions or lack of ability (due to an impairment) to perform an activity within the range considered normal, i.e. **activities that cannot be done**.
- **Handicap**—a limitation of normal occupation because of impairment or disability, i.e. **social consequences**.

    Thus:
    - **A hemiparesis is an impairment.**
    - **An inability to wash or dress is a disability.**
    - **An inability to do an occupation is a handicap.**

The introductory clinical training in the first few chapters of this book concentrates on evaluation of impairments. Disability and handicap are not always given due attention and are the practical and social aspects of the disease process. It is a mistake if the doctor is preoccupied by impairments, since the patient often perceives disability as the major problem.

The impairments, disability and handicap should have been covered in a normal history and examination, but it can be helpful to bring together important facts to provide an overall assessment.

A summary description of a patient may include the following.

- **Aetiology**—familial hypercholesterolaemia.
- **Pathology**
    - atheroma
    - right middle cerebral artery thrombosis
- **Impairment**
    - left hemiparesis
    - paralysed left arm, fixed in flexion
    - upper motor neuron signs in left arm and face
- **Disability**—difficulty during feeding. Cannot drive his car.
- **Handicap**
    - can no longer work as a travelling salesman
    - embarrassed to socialize
- **Social circumstances**—partner can cope with day-to-day living, but lack of income from his occupation and withdrawal from society present major problems.

Assessment of impairment

The routine history and examination will often reveal impairments. Additional standard clinical measures are often used to assist quantitation, e.g.

- treadmill exercise test
- peak flowmeter
- Medical Research Council scale of muscle power

— making five-pointed star from matches (to detect dyspraxia in hepatic encephalopathy)

Questionnaires can similarly provide a semiquantitative index of important aspects of impairment and give a brief short-hand description of a patient. The role of the questionnaire is in part a checklist to make sure the key questions are asked.

Cognitive function

In the elderly, impaired cognitive function can be assessed by a standard 10-point **mental test score** introduced by Hodkinson. The test assumes normal communication skills. One mark each is given for correct answers to 10 standard questions (**see Appendix 3 for questionnaire**):

— age of patient
— time (to nearest hour)
— address given, for recall at end of test, e.g. 42 West Street or 92 Columbia Road
— recognize two people
— year (if January, the previous year is accepted)
— name of place, e.g. hospital or area of town if at home
— date of birth of patient
— start of First World War
— name of monarch in UK, president in USA
— count backwards from 20 to 1 (no errors allowed unless self-corrected)
— (check recall of address)

This scale is a basic test of gross defects of memory and orientation and is designed to detect cognitive impairment. It has the advantages of brevity, relative lack of culture-specific knowledge and widespread use. In the elderly, 8–10 is normal, 7 is probably normal, 6 or less is abnormal.

Specific problems, such as confusion or wandering at night, are not included in the mental test score, and indicate that the score is a useful checklist but not a substitute for a clinical assessment.

Affect and drive

Motivation is an important determinant of successful rehabilitation. Depression, accompanied by lack of motivation, is a major cause of disability.

Enquire about symptoms of depression (p.16) and relevant examination (pp. 102 and 115), e.g. 'How is your mood? Have you lost interest in things?'

Making appropriate lifestyle changes, recruiting help from friends or relatives, can be key to increasing motivation. Pharmaceutical treatment of depression can also be helpful.

Assessment of disability

Assessing restrictions to daily activities is often the key to successful management.

O Make a list of disabilities separate from other problems, e.g. diagnoses, symptoms, impairments, social problems.

This list can assist with setting priorities, including which investigations or therapies are most likely to be of benefit to the patient.

Activities of daily living (ADL)

These are key functions which in the elderly affect the degree of independence. Several scales of disability have been used. One of these, the **Barthel index of ADL**, records the following disabilities that can affect self-care and mobility (see Appendix 4 for questionnaire):

— continence—urinary and faecal
— ability to use toilet
— grooming
— feeding
— dressing
— bathing
— transfer, e.g. chair to bed
— walking
— using stairs

The assessment denotes the current state and not the underlying cause or the potential improvement. It does not include cognitive functions or emotional state. It emphasizes independence, so a catheterized patient who can competently manage the device achieves the full score for urinary incontinence. The total score provides an overall estimate or summary of dependence, but between-patient comparisons are difficult as they may have different combinations of disability. Interpretation of score depends on disability and facilties available.

Instrumental activities of daily living (IADL)

These are slightly more complex activities relating to an individual's ability to live independently. They often require special assessment in the home environment.

- preparing a meal
- doing light housework
- using transport
- managing money
- shopping
- doing laundry
- taking medications
- using a telephone

Communication

In the elderly, difficulty in communication is a frequent problem, and impairment of the following may need special attention:

- deafness (do the ears need syringing? Is a hearing aid required?)
- speech (is dysarthria due to lack of teeth?)
- an alarm to call for help when required
- aids for reading, e.g. spectacles, magnifying glass
- resiting or adaptation of doorbell, telephone, radio or television

Analysing disabilities and handicaps and setting objectives

After writing a list of disabilities, it is necessary to make a possible treatment plan with specific objectives. The plan needs to be realistic. A multidisciplinary team approach, including

social workers, physiotherapists, occupational therapists, nurses and doctors is usually essential in rehabilitation of elderly patients.

The overall aims in treating the elderly include the following:

- To make diagnoses, if feasible, particularly to treatable illnesses.
- To comfort and alleviate problems and stresses, even if one cannot cure.
- To add life to years, even if one cannot add years to life.

Specific aspects which may need attention include the following:

- Alleviate social problems if feasible.
- Improve heating, clothing, toilet facilities, cooking facilities.
- Arrange support services, e.g. help with shopping, provision of meals, attendance to day centre.
- Arrange regular visits from nurse or other helper.
- Make sure family, neighbours and friends understand the situation.
- Treat depression.
- Help with sorting out finances.
- Provide aids, e.g.
  - large-handled implements
  - walking frame or stick
  - slip-on shoes
  - handles by bath or toilet
- Help to keep as mobile as feasible.
- Facilitate visits to hearing-aid centre, optician, chiropodist, dentist.
- Ensure medications are kept to a minimum, and the instructions and packaging are suitable.

A major problem is if the disability leads to the patient being unwelcome. This depends on the reactions of others and requires tactful discussion with all concerned.

Identifying causes for disabilities

Specific disabilities may have specific causes which can be alleviated. In the elderly, common problems include the following.

Confusion

This is an impairment. Common causes are:

- infection
- drugs
- other illnesses, e.g. heart failure
- sensory deprivation, e.g. deafness, darkness

Assume all confusion is an acute response to an unidentified cause.

Incontinence

- toilet far away, e.g. upstairs
- physical restriction of gait
- urine infection
- faecal impaction
- uterine prolapse
- diabetes

'Off legs'

- neurological impairment
- unsuspected fracture of leg
- depressed
- general illness, e.g. infection, heart failure, renal failure, hypothermia, hypothyroid, diabetes, hypokalaemia

Falls

- insecure carpet
- dark stairs
- poor vision, e.g. cataracts
- postural hypotension
- cardiac arrhythmias
- epilepsy
- neurological deficit, e.g. Parkinson's disease, hemiparesis
- cough or micturition syncope
- intoxication

CHAPTER 9

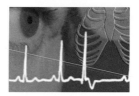

Basic Examination, Notes and Diagnostic Principles

Basic examination

In practice, one cannot attempt to elicit every single physical sign for each system. Basic signs should be sought on every examination, and if there is any hint of abnormality, additional physical signs can be elicited to confirm the suspicion. Listed below are the basic examinations of the systems which will enable you to complete a routine examination adequately but not excessively.

O **General examination**
- general appearance
- is the patient well or ill?
- look at temperature chart or take patient's temperature
- any obvious abnormality?
- mental state, mood, behaviour

O **General and cardiovascular system**
- observation—dyspnoea, distress
- blood pressure
- hands
    - temperature
    - nails, e.g. clubbing, liver palms
- pulse—rate, rhythm, character
- axillae—lymph nodes
- neck—lymph nodes
- face and eyes—anaemia, jaundice
- tongue and fauces—central cyanosis
- jugular venous pressure (JVP)—height and waveform
- apex beat—position and character
- parasternal—heave or thrills

- stethoscope
  - heart sounds, added sounds, murmurs
  - listen in all four areas with stethoscope diaphragm
  - lie patient on left side, bell of stethoscope—mitral stenosis (MS)
  - sit patient up, lean forward, breathe out—aortic incompetence (AI)
- **Respiratory system**
  - observation
  - trachea—position
  - **front of chest**
    - movement
    - percuss—compare sides
    - auscultate
  - **back of chest**
    - movement
    - percuss—particularly level of bases
    - auscultate
  - examine sputum
- **Examine spine.**
- **Abdomen**
  - lie patient flat
  - feel femoral pulses and inguinal lymph nodes
  - herniae
  - look at abdomen—ask if pain or tenderness
  - palpate abdomen gently
    - generally all over? masses
    - liver—then percuss
    - spleen—then percuss
    - kidneys
    - (ascites if indicated)
  - (auscultate if indicated)
  - males—genitals
  - per rectum (PR; only if given permission)—usually at end of examination
  - per vaginam (PV)—rarely by student

o **Legs**
  - observation
  - arterial pulses (joints if indicated)
  - neurology:
    - reflexes — knees   tone   ⎫
              — ankles   power   ⎬ only
              — plantar responses coordination ⎭ if indicated
    - sensation — pinprick   position   ⎫
              — vibration   cotton-wool ⎬ only
                                   temperature ⎭ if indicated

o **Arms**
  - posture: outstretched hands, eyes closed, rapid finger movements
  - finger–nose coordination:
    - reflexes — triceps   tone   ⎫
              — biceps   power   ⎬ only
              — supinator   ⎭ if indicated
    - sensation — pinprick   vibration   ⎫
                                   position   ⎪
                                   cotton-wool ⎬ only
                                   temperature ⎭ if indicated

o **Cranial nerves**
  - I (if indicated)
  - II: eyes — reading print
              — pupils — torch and accommodation
              — ophthalmoscope — fundi
              — fields
  - III, IV, VI: eye movements — 'Do you see double?'
              note nystagmus
  - V, VII — open mouth
              — grit teeth — feel masseters
              — sensation — cotton-wool
              — (corneal reflex — if indicated)
              — (taste — if indicated)
  - VIII: hearing — watch at each ear
      — (Rinne, Weber tests if indicated)
  - IX, X: fauces movement

- XI: shrug shoulders
- XII: put out tongue

o **Walk** — look at gait.
o **Herniae and varicose veins.**

Example of notes

Patient's name: **Age:**   **Occupation:**
State your name and designation, e.g. A. Bloggs SHO medicine
Date of admission:
Complains of:
- list, in patient's words

History of present illness:
- detailed description of each symptom (even if appears irrelevant)
- last well
- chronological order, with both actual date of onset, and time previous to admission
- (may include history from informant — in which case, state this is so)
- then detail other questions which seem relevant to possible differential diagnoses
- then **functional enquiry**, 'check' system for other symptoms
- (minimal statement in notes — weight, appetite, digestion, bowels, micturition, menstruation, if appropriate)

Past history:
- chronological order

Family history:

Personal and social history:
- must include details of home circumstances, dependants, patient's occupation
- effect of illness on life and its relevance to foreseeable discharge of patient
- smoking, alcohol, drug misuse, medications

Physical examination:
- general appearance, etc.
- then record findings according to systems

Minimal statement:

Healthy, well-nourished woman.

Afebrile, not anaemic, icteric or cyanosed.

No enlargement of lymph nodes.

No clubbing.

Breasts and thyroid normal.

Cardiovascular system (CVS):	Blood pressure, pulse rate and rhythm.
	JVP not raised.
	Apex position.
	Heart sounds 1 and 2, no murmurs.
Respiratory system:	Chest and movements normal.
	Percussion note normal.
	Breath sounds vesicular.
	No other sounds.
Abdominal system:	Tongue and fauces normal.
	Abdomen normal, no tenderness.
	Liver, spleen, kidneys, bladder impalpable.
	No masses felt.
	Hernial orifices normal.
	Rectal examination normal.
	Vaginal examination not performed.
	Testes normal.
Central nervous system (CNS):	Alert and intelligent.
	Pupils equal, regular, react equally to light and accommodation.
	Fundi normal.
	Normal eye movements.
	Other cranial nerves normal.
	Limbs normal.

Biceps jerks	+	+
Triceps jerks	+	+
Supinator jerk	+	+
Knee jerks	+	+
Ankle jerks	+	+

Plantar reflexes   ↓   ↓
Touch and vibration normal.
Spine and joints normal.
Gait normal.

Pulses (including dorsalis pedis and posterior tibial) palpable.

Summary

Write a few sentences only:
- — salient positive features of history and examination
- — relevant negative information
- — home circumstances
- — patient's medical state
  - — understanding of illness
  - — specific concerns

Problem list and diagnoses

After your history and examination, **make a list of**:
- — **the diagnoses you have been able to make**
- — **problems or abnormal findings which need explaining**

For example:
- — symptoms or signs
- — anxiety
- — poor social background
- — laboratory results
- — drug sensitivities

It is best to separate the current problems of actual or potential clinical significance requiring treatment or follow-up, from the inactive problems. An example is:

Active problems	Date
1 Unexplained episodes of fainting	1 week
2 Angina	since 1990
3 Hypertension—blood pressure 190/100 mmHg	1990
4 Chronic renal failure—plasma creatinine 200 μmol/l	August 1996
5 Widower, unemployed, lives on own	

6 Anxious about possibility of being injured in a fall
7 Smokes 40 cigarettes per day

Inactive problems	Date
1 Thyrotoxicosis treated by partial thyroidectomy	1976
2 ACE inhibitor-induced cough	1991

At first you will have difficulty knowing which problems to put down separately, and which can be covered under one diagnosis and a single entry. It is therefore advisable to rewrite the problem list if a problem resolves or can be explained by a diagnosis. When you have some experience, it will be appropriate to fill out the problems on a complete problem list at the front of the notes:

Active problems Include symptoms, signs, unexplained abnormal investigations, social and psychiatric problems	Date	Inactive problems Include major past illness, operation or hypersensitivities. Do not include problems requiring active care	Date

From the problem list, you should be able to make:
o **differential diagnoses**, including that which you think is most likely. Remember:
  – **common diseases occur commonly**
  – **an unusual manifestation of a common disease** is more likely than an uncommon disease
    – when you hear hoof beats, think of horses, not zebras
  – **do not necessarily be put off by some aspect which does not fit.** (What is the farmer's friend which has four legs, wags its tail and says 'cockadoodledoo'? A dog, and the sound was from another animal)
o **possible diagnostic investigations** you feel are appropriate
o **management and therapy** you think are appropriate
o **prognostic implications**

Diagnoses

The diagnostic terms which physicians use often relate to different levels of understanding:

Disordered function	Imobile painful joint	Breathlessness	Angina
	↑	↑	↑
Structural lesion	Osteoarthritis	Anaemia	Narrow coronary artery
	↑	↑	↑
Pathology	Iron-deposition fibrosis (haemochromatosis)	Iron deficiency	Aortitis
	↑	↑	↑
Aetiology	Inherited disorder of iron metabolism— homozygous for C282Y with A-H	Bleeding duodenal ulcer	*Treponema pallidum* (syphilis)

Different problems require diagnoses at different levels, which may change as further information becomes available. Thus, a patient on admission may be diagnosed as *pyrexia of unknown origin*. After a plain X-ray of the abdomen, he may be found to have a *renal mass* which on a computed tomographic (CT) scan becomes *perinephric abscess*, which from blood cultures is found to be *Staphylococcus aureus* infection. For a complete diagnosis all aspects should be known, but often this is not possible.

Note many terms are used as a diagnosis but, in fact, cover considerable ignorance, e.g. *diabetes mellitus* (originally 'sweet-tasting urine', but now also diagnosed by high plasma glucose) is no more than a descriptive term of disordered function. *Sarcoid* relates to a pattern of symptoms and a pathology of non-caseating granulomata, of which the aetiology is unknown.

Progress notes

While the patient is in hospital, full progress notes should be kept to give a complete picture of:

- how the diagnosis was established
- how the patient was treated
- the evolution of the illness
- any complications that occured

These notes are as important as the account of the original examination. In acute cases, record daily changes in signs and symptoms. In chronic cases, the relevant systems should be re-examined at least once a week and the findings recorded.

It is useful to separate different aspects of the illness:

- symptoms
- signs
- laboratory investigations
- general assessment, e.g. apparent response to therapy
- further plans, which would include educating the patient and his family about the illness.

Objective findings such as alterations in weight, improvement in colour, pulse, character of respirations or fluid intake and output are more valuable than purely **subjective statements** such as 'feeling better' or 'slept well'.

When appropriate, daily blood pressure readings or analyses of the urine should be recorded.

An account of all ward procedures such as aspirations of chest should be included.

Specifically record:

- the findings and comments of the physician or surgeon in charge
- results of a case conference
- an opinion from another department

Problem-oriented records

Dr Larry Weed proposed a system of note-keeping in which the history and examination constituted a database. All subsequent notes are structured according to the **specific numbered problems** in a problem list.

Problem-oriented records really require a special system of note-keeping. The full system is therefore not often used, but the problem list is an extremely valuable check that all aspects of the patient's illness are being covered.

Serial investigations

The results of these should be collected together in a **table** on a special sheet. When any large series of investigations is made, e.g. serial blood counts, erythrocyte sedimentation rates or multiple biochemical analyses, the results can also be expressed by a **graph**.

Operation notes

In patients undergoing surgical treatment, an operation note must be written immediately after the operation. Do not trust your memory for any length of time as several similar problems may be operated on at one session. Even if you are distracted by an emergency, the notes must be written up the same day as the operation. These notes should contain definite statements on the following facts:

- name of surgeon performing the operation and his assistant
- name of anaesthetist and anaesthetic used
- type and dimension of incision used
- pathological condition found, and mention of anatomical variations
- operative procedures carried out
- method of repair of wound and suture materials used
- whether drainage used, material used, and whether sutured to wound
- type of dressing used

Postoperative notes

Within the first 2 days after an operation note:

- the general condition of the patient
- any complication or troublesome symptom, e.g. pain, haemorrhage, vomiting, distension, etc.
- any treatment

Discharge note

A full statement of the patient's condition on discharge should be written:

- final diagnosis
- active problems
- medication and other therapies
- plan
- specific follow-up points, e.g. persistent depressive disorder, blood pressure monitoring
- what the patient has been told
- where the patient has gone, and what help is available
- when the patient is next being seen
- an estimate of the prognosis

If the patient dies, the student must attend a post-mortem and then complete his note by a short account of the autopsy findings.

CHAPTER 10

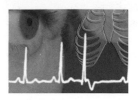

Presenting Cases and Communication

Presentations to doctors

Medicine is a subject in which you have to be able to talk. The more practice you get, the better you will become and the more confident you will appear in front of doctors, nurses and patients. Confidence displayed by the doctor is an important aspect of therapy and the value to the patient of a doctor who can speak lucidly is enormous.

Practise talking to yourself in a mirror, avoiding any breaks or interpolating the word 'er'. Open a textbook, find a subject and give a little talk on it to yourself. Even if you do not know anything about the subject, you will be able to make up a few coherent sentences once you are practised.

A presentation is not the time to demonstrate you have been thorough and have asked all questions, but is a time to show you can intelligently assemble the essential facts.

In all presentations, give the salient positive findings and the relevant negative findings.

For example:

— In a patient with progressive dyspnoea, state if patient has ever smoked.
— In a patient with icterus, state if patient has not been abroad, has not had any recent injections or drugs, or contact with other jaundiced patients.

Three types of presentations are likely to be encountered: presentation of a case to a meeting, presentation of a new case on a ward round and a brief follow-up presentation.

Presentation of a case to a meeting

This must be properly prepared, including visual aids as necessary. The principal details, shown on an overhead projector, are helpful as a reminder to you, and the audience may more easily remember the details of a case if they 'see' as well as 'hear' them.

- Practise your presentation from beginning to end and leave nothing to chance.
- Do not speak to the screen; speak to the audience.
- Do not crack jokes, unless you are confident that they are apposite.
- Do not make sweeping statements.
- Remember what you are advised to do in a court of law — dress up, stand up, speak up, shut up.
- Read up about the disease or problem beforehand so that you can answer any queries.
- Read a recent leading article, review or research publication on the subject.

In many hospitals it is expected that you present an **apposite, original article**. Be prepared to evaluate and criticize the manuscript. If your seniors cannot give you references, look up the subject on the internet or in large textbooks, or ask the always helpful librarian for advice. Laboriously repeating standard information from a textbook is often a turn-off. A recent series or research paper is more educational for you, and more interesting for the audience.

The overhead should summarizes any presentation:

Mr A.B.   Age: *x* years   Brief description, e.g. occupation

Complains of
(state in patient's words — for *x* period)

History of present complaint
- essential details
- other relevant information, e.g. risk factors
- relevant negative information relating to possible diagnoses
- extent to which symptoms or disease limit normal activity
- other symptoms — mention briefly

Past history
- briefly mention inactive problems
- information about active problems, or inactive problems relevant to present illness
- record allergies, including type of reaction to drugs

Family history
- brief information about parents, otherwise detail only if relevant

Social history
- brief unless relevant
- give family social background
- occupation and previous occupations
- any other special problems
- tobacco or ethanol abuse, past or present

Treatment
- note all drugs with doses

On examination

General description
- introductory descriptive sentence, e.g. well, obese man
- clinical signs relevant to disease
- relevant negative findings
  Remember these findings should be descriptive data rather than your interpretation.

Problem list

Differential diagnoses
(put in order of likelihood)

Investigations
- relevant positive findings
- relevant negative findings
- tables or graphs for repetitive data

— photocopy an electrocardiogram or temperature chart for overhead presentation

Progress report

Plan

Subjects which often are discussed after your presentation are:
- other differential diagnoses
- other features of presumed diagnosis that might have been present or require investigation
- pathophysiological mechanisms
- mechanisms of action of drugs and possible side-effects

After clinical discussion, be prepared to present a publication with essential details on an overhead.

Presentation of a new case on a ward round

- Good written notes are of great assistance. Do not read your notes word for word — use your notes as a reference.
- Highlight, underline or asterisk key features you wish to refer to, or write up a separate note-card for reference.
- Talk formally and avoid speaking too quickly or too slowly. Speak to the whole assembled group rather than a tête-à-tête with the consultant.
- Stand upright — it helps to make you appear confident.
- If you are interrupted by a discussion, note where you are and be ready to resume, repeating the last sentence before proceeding.

History

The format will be similar to that on an overhead, with emphasis on positive findings and relevant negative information. A full description of the initial main symptom is usually required.

Examination

Once your history is complete the consultant may ask for the relevant clinical signs only. Still add in relevant negative signs you think are important.

Summary

Be prepared to give a problem list and differential diagnoses.

If you are presenting the patient at the bedside, ensure the patient is comfortable. If the patient wishes to make an additional point or clarification, it is best to welcome this. If it is relevant it can be helpful. If irrelevant, politely say to the patient you will come back to him in a moment, after you have presented the findings. Do not appear to argue with the patient.

Brief follow-up presentation

Give a brief, orienting introduction to provide a framework on which other information can be placed. For example:

A *xx*-year-old man who was admitted *xx* days ago.

Long-standing problems include *xxxxx* (list briefly).

Presented with *xx* symptoms for *x* period.

On examination had *xx* signs.

Initial diagnosis of *xx* was confirmed/supported by/not supported by *xx* investigations.

He was treated by *xx*.

Since then *xx* progress:

— symptoms
— examination

Start with general description and temperature chart and, if relevant, investigations.

If there are multiple active problems, describe each separately, e.g.

— first in regard to the *xxxx*
— second in regard to the *xxxx*

The outstanding problems are *xxxx*.

The plan is *xxxx*.

Aide-mémoires

These are basic lists that provide brief reminders when presenting patients and diseases. Organizing one's thoughts along structured lines is helpful.

History

- principal symptom(s)
- history of present illness: 'How did your illness begin?'
- note chronology
- present situation
- functional enquiry
- past history
- family history
- personal and social history

Pain or other symptoms

- site
- radiation
- character
- severity
- onset/duration
- frequency/periodicity or constant
- precipitating factors
- relieving factors
- associated symptoms
- getting worse or better?

Lumps

Inspection

- site
- size
- shape
- surface
- surroundings

Palpation

- soft/solid consistency
- surroundings — fixed/mobile
- tender
- pulsatility
- transmission of illumination

Local lymph nodes

'Tell me about the disease'
- incidence
- geographical area
- gender/age
- aetiology
- pathology
  - macroscopic
  - microscopic
- pathophysiology
- symptoms
- signs
- therapy
- prognosis

Causes of disease
○ **genetic**
○ **infective**
- virus
- bacterial
- fungal
- parasitic

○ **neoplastic**
- cancer
  - primary
  - secondary
- lymphoma

○ **vascular**
- atheroma
- hypertension
- other, e.g. arteritis

○ **infiltrative**
- fibrosis
- amyloid
- granuloma

- autoimmune
- endocrine
- degenerative
- environmental
  - trauma
  - iatrogenic—drug side-effects
  - poisoning
- malnutrition
  - general
  - specific, e.g. vitamin defiency
  - perinatal with effects on subsequent development

Diagnostic labels

- aetiology, e.g. tuberculosis, genetic
  ↓
- pathology, e.g. sarcoid, amyloid
  ↓
- disordered function, e.g. hypertension, diabetes
  ↓
- symptoms or signs, e.g. jaundice, erythema nodosum

People—including patients

A significant number of disasters, a great deal of irritation and a lot of unpleasantness could be avoided in hospitals by proper communication. The doctor is not the boss but is part of a team, all of whom significantly help the patient. You must be able to communicate properly with the nursing staff, physiotherapists, occupational therapists, administrators, ancillary staff and, above all, patients.

When you first arrive on the wards it is a good idea to go and see the ward sister, physiotherapist, etc. and find out what their job is, what their difficulties are and how they view the patient, other groups and, most importantly, yourself.

Remember these points.

- **Time**—when you talk to anyone, try not to appear in a rush or they will lose concentration and not listen. A little time taken to talk to somebody properly will help enormously. One minute spent sitting down can seem like 5 minutes to the patient; 5 minutes standing up can seem like 1 minute.

o **Silence**—in normal social interaction we tend to avoid silences. In a conversation, as soon as one person stops talking (or even before) the other person jumps in to say his or her bit. When interviewing patients, it is often useful, if you wish to encourage the patient to talk further, to remain silent a moment longer than would be natural. An encouraging nod of the head, or an echoing of the patient's last word or two may also encourage the patient to talk further.

o **Listen**—active listening to someone is not easy but is essential for good communication. Many people stop talking but not all appear to be listening. Sitting down with the patient is advantageous, both in helping you to concentrate and in transmitting to the patient that you are willing to listen.

o **Smile**—grumpiness or irritation is the best way to stop a patient talking. A smile will often encourage a patient to tell you problems he would not normally do. It helps everybody to relax.

o **Reassurance**—if you appear confident and relaxed this helps others to feel the same. Being calm without excessive body movements can help. Note how a good consultant has a reassuring word for patients and allows others in the team to feel they are (or are capable of) working effectively. As a student you are not in a position to do this, but you can contribute by playing your role efficiently and calmly.

o **Humility**—no one, in particular the patient, is inferior to you.

CHAPTER 11

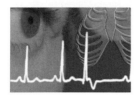

Imaging Techniques and Clinical Investigations

Introduction

This brief introduction to major clinical investigations starts with a general description of the major techniques, and is followed by specialized investigations in cardiology (see p. 199, with ECG p. 235), respiratory medicine (see p. 209), gastroenterology (see p. 214), renal medicine (see p. 217), neurology (see p. 218), haematology (see p. 220), biochemistry (see p. 225) and taking blood samples (see p. 230).

Ultrasound examinations

High-frequency (2.5–10 MHz) ultrasound waves are produced by the piezoelectric effect within ultrasound transducers. These transducers, which both produce and receive sound waves, are moved over the skin surface and images of the underlying organ structures are produced from the reflected sound waves. Structures with very few interfaces, such as fluid-filled structures, allow through transmission of the sound waves and therefore appear more **black** on the screen. Structures with a large number of interfaces cause significant reflection and refraction of the sound waves and therefore appear **whiter**. Air causes almost complete attenuation of the sound wave and therefore structures deep to this cannot be visualized.

Ultrasound scanning is a real-time examination and is dependent on the experience of the operator for its accuracy. The diagnosis is made from the real-time examination, although a permanent record of findings can be recorded on X-ray-like film.

The technique has the advantage of being safe, using non-ionizing radiation, being repeatable, painless and requiring little, if any, pre-preparation of the patient. It is also possible to carry out the examination at the patient's bedside and to evaluate a series of organs in a relatively short period of time.

Ultrasound is used in many different situations, including the following.

Abdomen
- **liver**—tumours, abscesses, diffuse liver disease, dilated bile ducts, hepatic vasculature
- **gallbladder**—gallstones, gallbladder wall pathology (Fig. 11.1)
- **pancreas**—tumours, pancreatitis
- **kidneys**—size, hydronephrosis, tumours, stones, scarring
- **spleen**—size, focal abnormalities
- **ovaries**—size, cysts, tumours
- **uterus**—pregnancy, tumours, endometrium
- **aorta**—aneurysm
- **bowel**—inflammation, tumours, abscesses

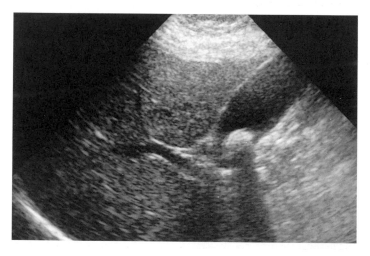

Fig. 11.1 Ultrasound scan showing a stone within gallbladder, casting an acoustic shadow.

Brain
- possible in the infant before the anterior fontanelle closes

Heart
See Echocardiography, p. 200.

Pleura
- pleural fluid or thickening

Blood vessels
- aneurysms, stenoses, clot in veins

Neck
- thyroid — characterization of masses

Scrotum
- tumours, inflammation

Musculoskeletal
- joint effusions, soft-tissue masses

Endoscopy

Internal organs are directly visualized, usually with a flexible fibreoptic endoscope.

Gastroscopy

A flexible scope is inserted by mouth after intravenous diazepam for direct vision of oesophagus, stomach and duodenum (see p. 214) (also see Endoscopic retrograde cholangiopancreatography (ERCP), p. 215).

Proctoscopy

With the patient lying in a left lateral position on one side, with knees and hips flexed, a short tube is introduced through the anus with a removable obturator lubricated with a gel. To investigate:
- **rectal bleeding** — haemorrhoids or anal carcinoma

Sigmoidoscopy

With the patient in left lateral position, either a rigid tube with a removable obturator or a flexible fibreoptic endoscope is introduced. Bowel is kept patent with air from a hand pump. To investigate:

— **bleeding, diarrhoea or constipation**—*ulcerative colitis*, other *inflammatory bowel disease* or *carcinoma*
— **inflamed area or lumps can be biopsied**

Colonoscopy

After the bowel is emptied with an oral purgative and a washout if necessary, the whole of the colon and possibly the terminal ileum can be examined. To investigate:

— **bleeding, diarrhoea or constipation**—*inflammatory bowel disease*, *polyps* or *carcinoma*

Bronchoscopy

After intravenous diazepam, the major bronchi are observed. To investigate:

— **haemoptysis or suspected bronchial obstruction**—*bronchial carcinoma* and for clearing *obstructed bronchi*, e.g. peanuts, plug of mucus

Laparoscopy

After general anaesthetic, organs can be observed through a small abdominal incision, aspirated for cells or organisms, or biopsied. Laparoscopic surgery includes sterilization, ova collection for *in vitro* fertilization and laparoscopic cholecystectomy.

Cystoscopy

After local anaesthetic, a cystoscope is inserted into the urethral meatus. To investigate:

— **urinary bleeding or poor flow**—*bladder tumours*
— under direct vision, catheters can be inserted into ureters for retrograde pyelograms

Colposcopy

Examination of cervix, usually to take a cervical smear. To investigate:

- **premalignant changes or cancer**

Needle biopsy

Core biopsy

A small core of tissue (30 × 1 mm) is obtained through needle puncture of organs for histological diagnosis. To investigate:

- liver — *cirrhosis, alcoholic liver disease, chronic active hepatitis*
- kidney — *glomerulonephritis, interstitial nephritis*
- lung — *fibrosis, tumours, tuberculosis*

Fine-needle aspiration

A technique to obtain cells for diagnosis of tumours or for microbiological diagnosis. The needle position is guided by ultrasound, computed tomographic (CT) scan or magnetic resonance imaging (MRI) scan. For investigation of many unexplained lumps, e.g. pancreas or breast lumps, to diagnose carcinoma.

Radiology

Conventional X-rays visualize only four basic radiographic densities: air, metal, fat and water. Air densities are black; metal densities (the most common of which are calcium and barium) are white with well-defined edges; fat and water densities are dark and mid grey.

There can be difficulty in visualizing a three-dimensional structure from a two-dimensional film. One helpful rule in deciding where a lesion is situated is to note which, if any, adjacent normal landmarks are obliterated. For example, a water density lesion which obliterates the right border of the heart must lie in the right middle lobe and not the lower lobe. A different view, e.g. lateral chest radiograph, is needed to be certain of the position of densities.

Chest radiograph

Use a systematic approach.

○ Posteroanterior (PA) or anteroposterior (AP) which are only done when the patient is in a bed (Fig. 11.2). The correct name for the usual chest study is 'a PA chest radiograph'. This means that the anteriorly situated heart is as close to the film as possible and its image will be minimally enlarged.

○ Follow a logical progression from centre of film to periphery
  — interfaces are only seen in silhouette when adjacent tissues have different 'stopping power' of X-rays. Thus heart border becomes invisible when collapse or consolidation in adjacent lung

○ **Technical factors**
  — positioning—apices and costophrenic angles should be on the film
  — inspiration—at least six posterior ribs seen above right diaphragm
  — penetration—mid cardiac intervertebral disc spaces visible
  — rotation—medial end clavicles equidistant from spinous processes
  — note any catheters, tubes, pacing wires, pneumothorax

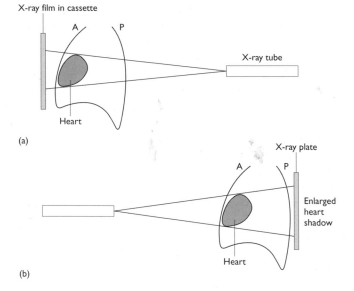

Fig. 11.2 (a) A normal posteroanterior (PA) X-ray; (b) an anteroposterior (AP) chest X-ray (mobile X-ray for chest radiographs of patients in bed).

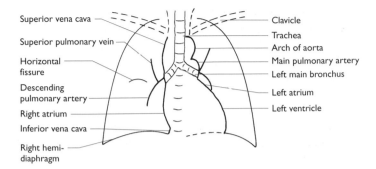

Fig. 11.3 Review particularly lungs, apices, costophrenic angles, hilar, behind heart.

o Heart
- — size
  - — normal <50% cardiothoracic ratio (maximum diameter heart ÷ maximum internal diameter of thoracic ribs as per cent)
  - — males <15.5 cm, females <15 cm diameter
- — shape—any chamber enlarged?
  - — PA radiograph: LV and RA
  - — lateral radiograph: RV and LA
- — calcification—in valves (better seen on lateral chest X-ray) or arteries

o Pericardium
- — globular suggests *pericardial infusion*
- — calcification suggests *tuberculosis*

o Aorta
- — large in aneurysms, small in *atrial septal defect*
- — calcification in intima, >6 mm inside outer wall suggests *dissection*

o Mediastinum
- — ? widening—look at lateral chest X-ray to locate

o Hila
- — right at horizontal fissure, left 0–2.5 cm higher
  - — displacement suggests loss of lung volume, e.g. *collapse, fibrosis*

- enlargement
  - if lobulated — a *mass or lymph nodes*
  - ? vascular dilation
- density — ? mass projected over hilum

○ **Pulmonary vessels**
- large in intracardiac or peripheral shunts — prominent in outer third (plethora)
- large in *pulmonary hypertension* with small vessels in outer third (pruning) — *shunts, hypoxia, emboli, chronic lung disease*
- segmental avascularity — *pulmonary emboli*
- small in *congenital heart disease, right ventricular/pulmonary artery atresia*

○ **Lung parenchyma**
- lungs should be equally transradiant (black)
- alveolar shadows — ill-defined or confluent and dense
  - air bronchogram — water, pus, blood, tumour around patent bronchi, often seen end on, as a circle, near hila
- nodular shadows, e.g. *granuloma, tuberculosis*
- reticular shadows — *fibrotic lung disease*
    Note uniformity, symmetry, unilateral or bilateral, upper or lower zones.
- masses
  - define position (ask for lateral chest radiograph), edge, shape, size
  - *tumour, abscess, embolus, infection*

○ **Pleura**
- fluid
  - homogeneous, opaque shadow, usually with lateral meniscus
  - if air–fluid interface, *empyema* or after thoracocentesis
- pneumothorax
  - peripheral space devoid of markings with edge of lung visible
  - look for mediastinal displacement — *tension pneumothorax*
- masses
  - lobulated shadows — loculated fluid or tumour

o **Skeleton**
  - sclerosis, focal—?*metastases, e.g. breast, prostate, stomach, kidney, thyroid, lymphoma*
       —*myelofibrosis, Paget's disease*
  - lytic—?*metastases, e.g. lung, colorectal, myeloma*
  - osteopenia (only visible when advanced)—osteoporosis and osteomalacia cannot be distinguished on radiographs, except Looser's zones (pseudofracture) in osteomalacia
  - look for fractures
o **Other areas**
  - hiatus hernia, behind heart
  - left lower lobe collapse, behind heart
  - lungs behind dome of diaphragm
  - gas below diaphragm on erect chest radiograph—*perforated viscus, recent surgery*
  - apices—? lung visible above clavicle

Abdominal radiography

This is less satisfactory than chest radiography because there are fewer contrasting densities. Air in the gut is helpful, as are the psoas lines. Try to find as many organ outlines as possible.

  - Supine (AP) radiograph—routine.
  - Erect radiograph
       - for air–fluid levels (AFLs)
           - <5 short AFLs normal
           - many—*obstruction*
           - also in *paralytic ileus, coeliac disease, jejunal diverticula*
o **Visceral organs**
  - liver

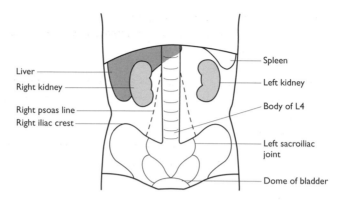

- usually <18 cm long—inferior surface outlined by fat
- ? gas in biliary tree centrally
- spleen—enlargement displaces stomach gas bubble to mid-line
- kidneys—normally 3–3.5 vertebrae long

○ **Bowel gas pattern**
  - stomach
    - normally small air bubble
    - dilated in *pyloric stenosis* and *proximal small-bowel obstruction*
  - small bowel
    - central position
    - small loops, valvulae across lumen, no faeces
    - dilated when >3.5 cm proximally, >2.5 cm distally—suggests *obstruction*
  - large bowel
    - vertical in flanks and across top of abdomen
    - wider loops, haustral folds do not cross lumen ± faeces
    - dilated when >5.5 cm—suggests obstruction
    - >9 cm—suggests perforation risk
  - hernial orifices—? bowel air pattern below femoral neck indicates herniae

○ **Abnormal gas**
  - pneumoperitoneum
  - both sides of bowel defined as thin lines

- loss of liver density from gas anteriorly
- bowel wall—thin streaks of gas suggest infarction or gas-producing bacteria

o Abnormal calcification
- 30% gallstones are radiopaque—can be anywhere in abdomen
- pancreas calcification—follows oblique line of pancreas and suggests *chronic pancreatitis*
- renal stones—usually radiopaque
- nephrocalcinosis—*medullary sponge kidney* or *metabolic calcinosis*
- in phleboliths or foecoliths in diverticulae

o Other soft tissues
- psoas lines
    - outlined by retroperitoneal fat
    - absent in 20% of normals
    - unilateral absence suggests *retroperitoneal mass* or *haematoma*
- ascites
    - uniformly grey appearance
    - bowel gas 'floats' centrally

Computed tomography

A segment of the body is X-rayed at numerous angles as the apparatus rotates through 360°. A computer summarizes the data from multiple pictures to provide a composite picture (Fig. 11.4). Attenuation of X-rays depends on tissue—water is arbitrary 0, black is −1000 and white is +1000 Hounsfield units. Different 'windows' are chosen to display different characteristics, e.g. soft-tissue window, lung window, bone window.
CT can be used:
- for organs and masses in abdomen and thorax
- to diagnose tumours, infarcts and bleeds in cerebral hemispheres
- for posterior fossa—lesions less easy to visualize because of bony base of skull
- to visualize disc prolapse and neoplasm in spinal cord, but adjacent bones interfere. Intrathecal contrast medium is often required for cord tumours

Variants of CT:
- intravenous contrast

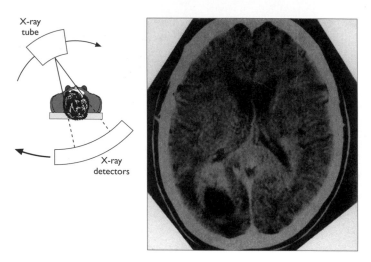

Fig. 11.4 Computed tomographic scan across cerebral hemispheres.

- iodine-based
- opacifies blood vessels
- shows leaky vessels or increased number of vessels
- oral contrast
  - opacifies gut contents
- spiral CT
  - X-ray tube constantly rotated with patient moving
  - computer segments into slices
  - advantages —faster, more detail, can use intravenous contrast medium
  - *becoming the investigation of choice for pulmonary embolism*

Arteriography and venography

An X-ray film is taken after a radiopaque contrast has been injected into a blood vessel (Fig. 11.5):

- coronary arteriography, e.g. *coronary artery disease*
- cerebral angiography, e.g. *aneurysm* after *subarachnoid haemorrhage*

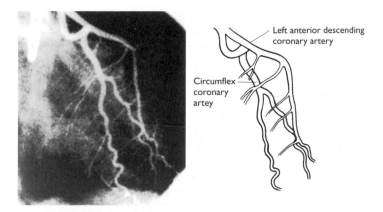

Fig. 11.5 Left coronary artery angiogram viewed from right.

- carotid angiography e.g. *stenoses*
- pulmonary angiography, e.g. *pulmonary embolus* or *fistula*
- renal angiography, e.g. *renal artery stenosis, arteriovenous fistula*
- aortography and iliofemoral angiography, e.g. *aortic aneurysm, iliofemoral artery atheroma*
- leg venogram, e.g. *deep venous thrombosis*

Concurrent venous blood sampling may help localize an endocrine tumour, e.g. parathormone from an occult parathyroid tumour, catecholamines from a phaeochromocytoma, or to confirm the significance of renal artery stenosis using renal vein renin analyses.

Background subtraction angiography

Contrast is inserted rapidly via a peripheral vein (intravenous digital subtraction angiography) or into the artery (intra-arterial subtraction angiography). As the contrast passes along the vessel concerned, X-ray pictures are taken.

In **digital subtraction** a computer subtracts the background field, leaving a clear view of the artery (Fig. 11.6):
- used to observe arterial stenoses or aneurysms
- can be used to assess left ventricular function

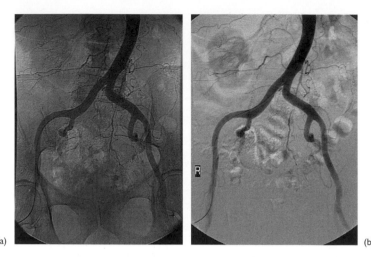

(a)   (b)

Fig. 11.6 Background subtraction angiography: (a) before; (b) after. Catheter inserted via right femoral artery. Contrast shows aorta and iliac arteries.

Nuclear medicine studies

These studies utilize radioactive isotopes (mostly technetium 99 m) coupled to appropriate pharmaceuticals or monoclonal antibodies designed to seek out different organ systems or pathology. The studies yield functional rather than morphological information. They are equisitely sensitive, but not specific.

> Lesions present either as photon-abundant areas (as in bone or brain) or photon-deficient areas (as in liver, lung, hearts, etc.).

The following are the commonest investigations routinely available.

Skeletal system

Any cause of increased bone turnover or altered blood flow to bone, e.g. tumour, infection, trauma, infarction. Used mostly for detection of metastases.

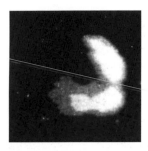
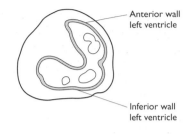

Anterior wall
left ventricle

Inferior wall
left ventricle

Fig. 11.7 Thallium 201 study of the heart.

Pulmonary system

The diagnosis of pulmonary emboli using perfusion scintigraphy, when emboli cause defects which do not correspond to water densities in the same position on simultaneous chest radiographs. Usually only indicated when chronic obstructive airways disease is present (see p. 213).

Cardiovascular system

For the measurement of ventricular function, e.g. ejection fractions, and for examining myocardial integrity. Ischaemia or scarring causes 'cold' areas on myocardial scintigrams. Studies are usually carried out at rest and after exercise (see p. 203).

Urogenital system

Renography (an activity–time curve of the passage of radioactive tracer through the kidney) for detecting abnormalities of renal blood flow, parenchymal function and excretion. Renal scintigraphy will detect scarring and is used to measure divided renal function. Chromium-51 EDTA (ethylene diamine tetra-acetic acid) clearance measurements yield accurate assessment of glomerular filtration rate. Methods are also available for detecting testicular torsion.

Cerebral scintigraphy

For the detection of abnormalities associated with certain neuro-psychiatric disorders, notably the dementias, schizophrenia and epilepsy.

Thyroid

For estimation of the size, shape and position of the gland, detecting the presence of 'hot' thyrotoxic nodules or 'cold' nodules caused by adenoma, carcinoma, cysts, haemorrhage or any combination thereof. Iodine uptake can also be estimated simultaneously.

Adrenals

The detection of autonomously functioning Conn's tumours (cortex) and phaechromocytoma (medulla).

Reticuloendothelial system

Mapping of the bone marrow and lymphatic flow. Occasionally used to visualize the liver and spleen if ultrasound not available.

In addition radiolabelled white cells can be used to search for infection or inflammation, notably in bone, suspected inflammatory bowel disease and after abdominal surgery.

Tracers are also available for detecting certain tumours, notably lymphoma, colonic carcinoma, ovarian carcinoma and malignant melanoma. Labelled red cells can detect sites of gastrointestinal bleeding. Oesophageal and gastric emptying studies are also available.

Magnetic resonance imaging

Also known as nuclear magnetic resonance (NMR). Provides cross-sectional images (MRI) or spectroscopic information on chemicals in tissues (magnetic resonance spectroscopy, MRS).

A small trolley carries the patient into a super-conducting magnet that provides a strong external magnetic field.

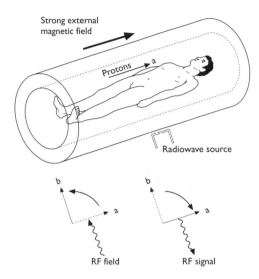

The axes of individual hydrogen ions usually lie at random but can be lined up at a particular angle by a strong magnetic field (position a). When subjected to a second radiofrequency magnetic field the angle is changed (to position b). When the radiowaves cease, position a is restored by the continuing magnetic field and a radiowave is emitted and detected.

Hydrogen MRI

Hydrogen is the most plentiful element in the body. MRI can detect differences between the concentration of hydrogen ions in different tissues, notably fat ($-CH2-$) and water (HOH).

Excellent for the examination of the head and spinal cord:

— the brain for demonstrating tumours, multiple areas of demyelination of white matter in multiple sclerosis (Fig. 11.8), spinal cord lesions, including disc prolapse
— bone and soft-tissue tumours

MRI will show detailed cross-sectional anatomical detail similar to CT scanning but can also provide coronal and sagittal planes in addition to the standard axial plane available from CT scanning.

Images can be obtained that accentuate different characteristics:

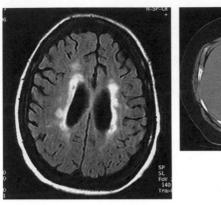

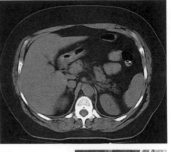

(a)

(b)

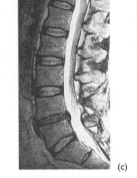

(c)

Fig. 11.8 (a) MRI T_1-weighted scan of the brain. The central white areas are areas of demyelination in multiple sclerosis and subcutaneous fat is white. (b) MRI T_2-weighted scan (sagittal section) of the abdomen showing the liver, top of the kidneys, spleen, pancreas, aorta with arterial branches and oral contrast in the jejunum. (c) MRI T_2-weighted scan (coronal section) of the lumbar spine showing white central spinal fluid surrounding the spinal cord.

- **spin echo T_1-weighted**
    - fat — white (bright)
    - fluid — dark
    - cortical bone — black
- **spin echo T_2-weighted**
    - fat — grey
    - fluid — white (bright)
- **gradient echo**
    - flowing blood — white
    - used for MRI angiography
- **intravenous contrast**
    - gadolinium-based
    - leaky vessels from inflammation

— increased number of vessels from neoplasm
— oral contrast—to label bowel

N.B. Patients with pacemakers should not be subjected to MRI. Patients with metal implants may not be able to undergo MRI and must be discussed with a radiologist. MRI has an expanding role in many fields of medicine and the indications are likely to increase.

PET scanning

Positron emmission tomography (PET) is imaging using 18-F-dioxyglucose (FDG). FDG uptake correlates with glucose metabolism. Malignant tumours actively metabolize glucose making it possible to image tumours using this technique. PET scanning needs futher evaluation but is likely to be useful in oncology.

Cardiological investigations

Electrocardiogram
See Chapter 12, p. 235.

Exercise electrocardiography (stress testing)

— Exercise may reveal cardiac dysfunction not apparent at rest.
— Most commonly used in suspected coronary artery disease.

Connected to a 12 lead electrocardiograph (ECG) machine, with resuscitation equipment available, the patient exercises at an increasing workload on a treadmill (or bicycle). **Bruce protocol**: 3-minute stages of increasing belt speed and treadmill gradient. Take ECG every minute, blood pressure every 3 minutes.

This assesses:
— exercise capacity
— haemodynamic response
— symptoms
— ECG changes

Exercise for as long as possible stopping when there are:
— marked symptoms
— severe ECG changes

- ventricular arrhythmias
- fall in blood pressure

Myocardial ischaemia causes ST segment depression. A high false-positive rate occurs in absence of angina (c. 20%). False-positive incidence depends on age and sex, with young females having the highest rate, even in the presence of typical symptoms of angina.

Clinically important abnormalities are:

- horizontal or downward sloping ST depression (Fig. 11.9)
- deep ST depression
- ST changes with typical anginal symptoms

A definitely negative test at a high workload denotes an excellent prognosis.

- **Angiography is indicated** if only a low workload is achieved before important abnormalities occur
- **Medical treatment of angina** may be appropriate if three or four stages are completed.

Echocardiography

This visualizes structures and function of the heart. Uses ultrasound (2.5–7.5 MHz) to reflect from interfaces in the heart, e.g. ventricle and atrial walls, heart, valves, major vessels. The higher frequency gives better discrimination but lower tissue penetration. The time delay between transmission and reception indicates depth.

Two-dimensional echocardiography

2D echocardiography (Fig. 11.10) uses a scanning beam swept backwards and forwards across a 45° or 60° arc to construct a picture of the anatomy of the heart.

2D echocardiography is excellent for demonstrating:

- valvular anatomy
- ventricular function, e.g. poor contraction, low ejection fraction, akinetic segment, paradoxical motion in aneurysm
- structural abnormalities:
  - pericardial effusion
  - ventricular hypertrophy
  - congenital heart disease

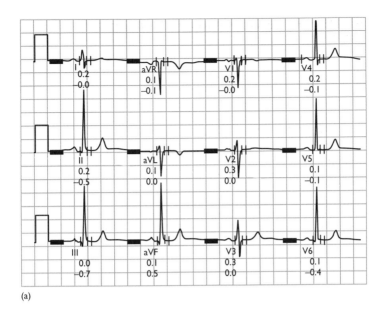

(a)

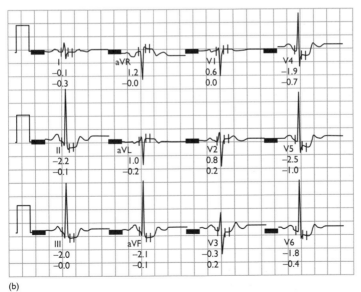

(b)

Fig. 11.9 Example of a strongly positive exercise test—signal averaged recordings before exercise (a) and at peak effort (b). There is a marked horizontal ST depression in the inferolateral leads, II, III, aVF and V4–6.

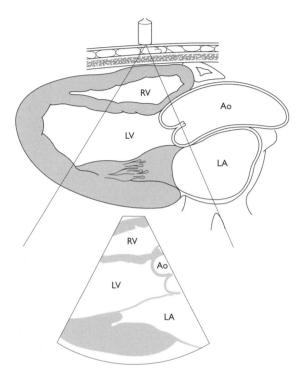

Fig. 11.10 Two-dimensional echocardiograph. Ao = aorta; LA = left atrium; LV = left ventricle; RV = right ventricle.

Quantifying valvular function is better achieved by Doppler echocardiography (see p. 204).

M-mode echocardiography

M-mode echocardiography (Fig. 11.11) uses a single pencil beam, and movements of the heart in that beam are visualized on moving sensitized paper. It predates 2D echocardiography but is useful for measuring ventricular diameters in systole/diastole.

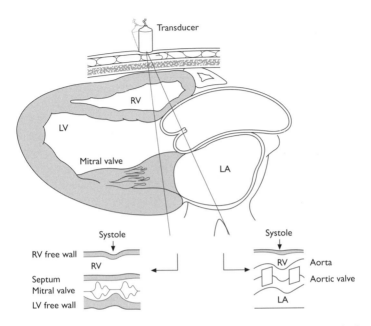

Fig. 11.11 M-mode echocardiographs, with two examples showing mitral and aortic valves opening and closing. LA = left atrium; LV = left ventricle; RV = right ventricle.

Radionuclide imaging in cardiology

Radionuclides can be used in the assessment of cardiac disease in three main ways.

Myocardial perfusion scintigraphy

- **Demonstrates abnormal blood flow in coronary artery disease** in conjunction with exercise testing. Thallium 201 is extracted from the blood in proportion to flow.
- Ischaemic myocardium appears as a cold spot on the scan taken immediately after injection of thallium.
- If the area is not infarcted, the cold spot 'fills in' as thallium redistributes in the following 4 hours.

— Thallium scanning is a more reliable diagnostic investigation than exercise testing and the number and extent of defects correlate with prognosis.

Radionuclide ventriculography (multiple gated acquisition (MUGA) scanning)

— Assesses ventricle function.

The patient's blood (usually red blood cells) is labelled with technetium 99 m (half-life 6 hours). A gamma camera and a computer generate a moving image of the heart by 'gating' the computer to the patient's ECG.

Systolic function of the left ventricle is quantified by the ejection fraction (normally 0.50–0.70):

$$\text{Ejection fraction} = \frac{\text{stroke volume}}{\text{end-diastolic volume}},$$

i.e. the proportion of the total diastolic volume that is ejected in systole.

Images can be collected during exercise as well as at rest, to assess the effect of stress on left ventricular function.

Pyrophosphate scanning

— Demonstrates recent myocardial infarction, e.g. 1–10 days after event.

Technetium 99 m pyrophosphate is taken up by areas of myocardial infarction producing a hot spot, maximal at 3 days.

Indicated when:

— the ECG is too abnormal to demonstrate infarction (e.g. left bundle-branch block)
— the patient has presented after the plasma enzyme changes, e.g. at 3 days

Doppler ultrasound cardiography

— Velocity of blood movement in the heart and circulation assessed by Doppler shift.

- Blood accelerates through an obstruction, e.g. a stenosed valve. The peak velocity is proportional to the haemodynamic gradient.
- Reverse flow pattern in valvular reflux.

Multigated Doppler or colour-flow Doppler

- Rapid method of detecting abnormal blood flow due to a leaking valve or an intracardiac shunt, e.g. ventricular septal defect.

Doppler ultrasound provides functional assessment to complement the anatomical assessment of 2D echocardiography.

- Echo machine calculates the direction and velocity of flow, pixel by pixel, within a segment of the image and codes it in colour.
- It superimposes flow on the 2D image.

Cardiac catheterization

An invasive assessment of cardiac function and disease in which fine tubes are passed, with mild sedation under operating theatre conditions:

- retrograde through arteries to left side of heart and coronary arteries
- anterograde through veins to right side of heart and pulmonary arteries
    - to make diagnosis, e.g. is valve critically stenosed?
    - is chest pain due to coronary artery disease?
    - to plan cardiac surgery, particularly coronary artery bypass grafting

It entails:

- a major radiation dose
    Major complications (one in 2000 cases) in:
    - access artery dissection (2%)
    - myocardial infarction (0.1%)
    - air or cholesterol emboli can cause stroke or myocardial infarction
    - death (0.01%)
- risks must be outweighed by the benefit the patient receives

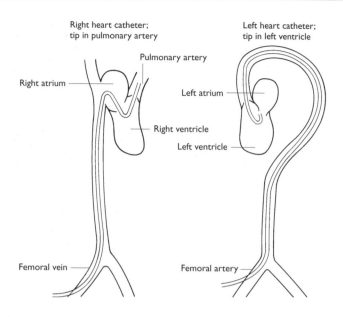

The commonest approach is **cannulation of the right femoral vessels by the Seldinger technique**. A percutaneous fine gauge needle punctures the vessel, through which a soft guide wire is passed. The needle is withdrawn and an introducer sheath and catheter is inserted over the guide wire which is then withdrawn. Haemostasis is achieved by compression. The technique is not suitable if the patient is on anticoagulant drugs, has severe peripheral vascular disease or an abdominal aortic aneurysm.

Alternative approach: **brachial vessels at elbow through a skin incision**. Closure of arterotomy by sutures allows use in anticoagulated patients.

Pressure measurements

Cardiac haemodynamics and gradients across individual valves, e.g. by pulling the catheter back across the **aortic valve**, whilst systolic pressures is recorded (Fig. 11.12).

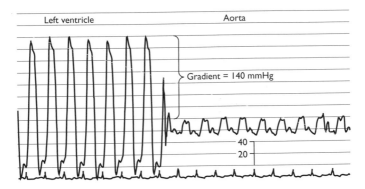

Fig. 11.12 Aortic stenosis. The systolic pressure falls as the catheter tip leaves the left ventricle, crossing the stenosed aortic valve. Diastolic pressure is prevented from falling by the aortic valve.

Mitral stenosis is quantified by the diastolic pressure difference between the left ventricle (**left heart catheter**) and left atrium measured indirectly via the **right heart catheter** in the 'wedge' position—passed through the pulmonary artery to occlude a pulmonary arteriole so the pressure at the tip reflects the left atrial pressure transmitted through the pulmonary capillaries (Fig. 11.13).

The **cardiac output** is calculated either by the **Fick principle** (cardiac output is inversely proportional to difference between systemic arterial and mixed venous blood oxygen saturation) or by the **thermodilution** technique.

Radio-opaque contrast

Radio-opaque contrast (iodine-based) is:
- injected into chambers to assess their systolic function and to detect valve regurgitation, e.g. left ventricular injection for mitral regurgitation
- injected into coronary ostia to detect coronary artery disease, with X-ray pictures multiple projections

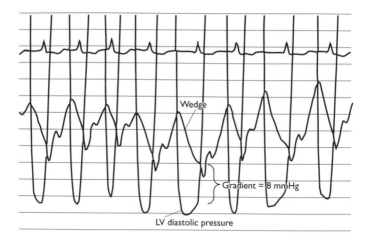

Fig. 11.13 Mitral stenosis. Left ventricular (LV) pressure trace expanded to show low diastolic pressures. A pressure difference between the wedge trace and LV diastolic trace reflects obstruction to flow into the left ventricle due to mitral stenosis. The rhythm is atrial fibrillation.

Twenty-four-hour ECG tape recording

ECG worn for 24 hours (or 48 hours) (Fig. 11.14); obtains on tape a continuous ECG recording during normal activities.

For diagnosis of:
- palpitations
- dizzy spells
- light-headedness or black-outs of possible cardiac origin

May show episodes of:
- atrial asystole
- atrial or ventricular tachycardias
- complete heart block
- ST segment changes during angina or silent ischaemia

Twenty-four-hour blood pressure recording

Blood pressure is measured intermittently with an upper arm cuff and

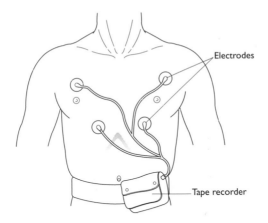

Fig. 11.14 Arrangement for the 24-hour ECG tape recorder.

microphone, with recording on a tape. Allows evaluation of blood pressure during everyday activities without the 'white coat' effect of anxiety at the doctor's surgery increasing measured blood pressure. Hypertension is defined as daytime average >140/>90 mmHg. Absence of lower blood pressure during the night ('dip') suggests secondary hypertension.

Respiratory investigations

pH and arterial blood gases

Normal ranges:
- pH 7.35–7.45
- P_{CO_2} 4.5–6.2pK$_a$
- P_{O_2} > 10.6pK$_a$
- HCO_3^- 22–26 mmol/l
- base excess is the amount of acid required to titrate pH to 7.4

In ventilatory failure:
- P_{O_2} low
- P_{CO_2} high

In respiratory failure from lung disease often:
- P_{O_2} low

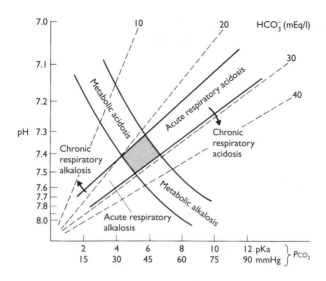

Fig. 11.15 Descriptive clinical terms. Shaded area is normal range.

— normal P_{CO_2} due to high carbon dioxide (CO_2) solubility and efficient transfer in lungs.

For example, in asthma, raised CO_2 signifies tiredness and decreased ventilation from reduced muscular effort.

Respiratory acidosis

CO_2 retention from:
— respiratory disease with right-to-left shunt
— ventilatory failure
    — neuromuscular disease
    — physical causes, e.g. flail chest, kyphoscoliosis
Raised CO_2 leads to increased bicarbonate:

$$CO_2 + H_2O = H_2CO_3 = H^+ + HCO_3^-.$$

In chronic respiratory failure, renal compensation by excretion of H^+ and retention of HCO_3^- leads to further increased HCO_3^-, i.e. maintenance of normal pH with compensatory metabolic alkalosis.

Respiratory alkalosis

CO_2 blown off by hyperventilation due to:

- hysteria
- brainstem stimulation (rare)

In respiratory alkalosis:

- Po_2 normal
- Pco_2 low

If chronic, compensated by metabolic acidosis with renal retention of H^+ and excretion of HCO_3^-.

Metabolic acidosis

Excess H^+ in blood:

- ketosis—3-OH butyric acid accumulation in diabetes or starvation
- uraemia—lack of renal H^+ excretion
- renal tubular acidosis—lack of H^+ or NH_4^- excretion
- acid ingestion—aspirin
- lactic acid accumulation—shock, hypoxia, exercise, biguanide
- formic acid accumulation—methanol intake
- loss of base—diarrhoea

Usually compensatory respiratory alkalosis, e.g. Kussmaul respiration of diabetic coma (hyerventilation with deep breathing):

- Po_2 normal
- Pco_2 low
- to assist diagnosis, measure anion gap

$$[Na^+] + [K^+] - [Cl^-] - [HCO_3^-] = 7{-}16\,mmol/l.$$

If anion gap >16 mmol/l, unestimated anions are present, e.g. 3-OH butyrate, lactate, formate.

Metabolic alkalosis

Loss of H^+ due to:

- prolonged vomiting
- potassium depletion—secondary to renal tubular potassium—hydrogen exchange

— ingestion of base—old-fashioned sodium bicarbonate therapy of peptic ulcers

Usually compensatory respiratory acidosis with hypoventilation:

— Po_2 low
— Pco_2 high

Peak flow

— Blow into machine as hard and fast as you can.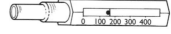
— Records in litres per minute. Useful for diagnosing and observing asthma. Normal range is 300–500 l/min.
— Improvement with β-agonist, e.g. isoprenaline, indicates reversible airway disease, i.e. asthma.

Spirometry

— Blow into machine, a **vitalograph**, as hard as you can—measures pattern of airflow during forced expiration.
— To distinguish between restrictive lung disease, e.g. *emphysema*, *fibrosis* and *obstructive lung disease*, e.g. *asthma, chronic obstructive airways disease.*

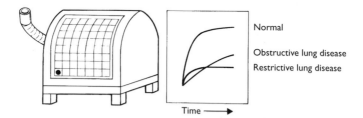

Normal

Obstructive lung disease
Restrictive lung disease

Time ⟶

Skin testing for allergens

Drops of a weak allergen solution are placed on to the skin, and a superficial prick of the skin, with a short lancet though the liquid, inoculates the epidermis. Special lancets coated with freeze-dried allergen can be used. A local wheal indicates an allergic response.

Carbon monoxide transfer factor

The rate of uptake of carbon monoxide from inspired gas determines the lung diffusion capacity. It is reduced in alveolar diseases, e.g. *pulmonary fibrosis*.

Ventilation/perfusion scan

Ventilation (V) scan
— Inhalation of an isotope allows picture of parenchyma of the lungs to be taken by a gamma camera.

Perfusion (P) scan
— Injection of isotope into the blood stream demonstrates the blood flow in the lungs.

> Mismatch of the scans is used to diagnose pulmonary embolism, i.e. air reaches all parts of the lung, while the blood does not (Fig. 11.16). Matching defects occur with other lung pathologies, e.g. *emphysema*.

N.B. A perfusion scan showing an area of ischaemia with a normal chest X-ray is generally sufficient to diagnose a pulmonary embolus. A *V/Q* scan is needed if there is other lung pathology suspected or on X-ray (e.g. chronic bronchitis/emphysema), but in practice the results are difficult to interpret.

Bronchoscopy

Flexible bronchoscopy—under mild sedation, e.g. intravenous diazepam with local anaesthetic spray to pharynx and larynx. Vision by fibreoptics.
— Obstructions can be visualized.
— Biopsies can be taken for neoplasms.
— Aspiration samples, sometimes after lavage with saline, can be taken for organisms and malignant cells.

Bronchogram—rarely done—a contrast medium is injected into the bronchial tree to show peripheral dilated bronchi (*bronchiectasis*).

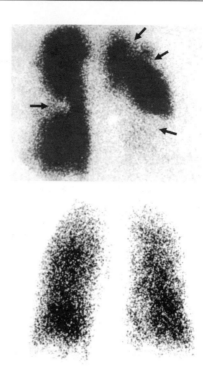

Fig. 11.16 V/Q scan of pulmonary embolism: (a) perfusion scan (arrows mark perfusion defects); (b) ventilation scan—normal.

Gastrointestinal investigations

Upper gastrointestinal endoscopy

A flexible fibreoptic tube is introduced into the oesophagus, stomach and duodenum after mild sedation, e.g. intravenous diazepam, with local anaesthetic to pharynx.

Direct vision of the gastrointestinal tract to investigate:
— **dysphagia**—oesophageal tumour or stricture
— **haematemasis or melaena**—oesophageal varices, gastric and duodenal ulcers, superficial gastric erosions, gastric carcinoma
— **epigastric pain**—peptic ulcer, oesophagitis, gastritis, duodenitis
— **unexplained weight loss**—gastric carcinoma

Endoscopic retrograde cholangiopancreatography

Through a fibreoptic endoscope, with a picture on a video, under direct vision, a tube is inserted through the ampulla of Vater at the opening of the common bile duct, and introduction of a radiopaque contrast medium allows X-ray visualization of:
— **biliary tree**, for stones, tumours, strictures, irregularities
— **pancreatic ducts**, for chronic pancreatitis, dilated ducts or distortion from a tumour

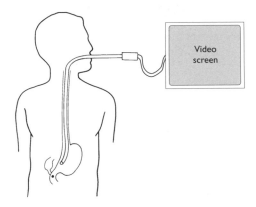

The endoscope can be used for surgery, including **sphincterotomy** of ampulla for removal of gallstones in the bile duct or the introduction of a rigid tube, **a stent**, through a constricting tumour to allow biliary drainage.

Proctoscopy, sigmoidoscopy, colonoscopy

See p. 183.

Barium swallow, meal, enema

Barium is drunk (swallow for oesophagus, meal for stomach/duodenum) or introduced rectally (enema) or via a catheter into the duodenum (small-bowel enema).

> X-rays are taken with barium coating the mucosa. Air may be introduced to distend organs and to give double-contrast films.

O It outlines physical abnormalities:
  - strictures, e.g. *fibrosis, carcinomata*
  - filling defects, e.g. *polyps, carcinomata*
  - craters, e.g. *ulcers, diverticula*
  - mucosal irregularities
    - mucosal folds radiating from *peptic ulcer*
    - clefts in *Crohn's disease of ileum and colon*
    - featureless mucosa of *early ulcerative colitis*
    - islands of mucosa in *severe ulcerative colitis*
      An irregularity on a single film needs to be seen on other views before an abnormality is confirmed, as peristalsis or gut contents can mimic defects.

Oral cholecystogram

This procedure is now rarely done as ultrasound is superior.

An initial plain film is taken to show radiopaque gallstones. A radiopaque contrast medium is taken by mouth, excreted by the liver and concentrated in the gallbladder.

  - Cholesterol gallstones give filling defects in the gallbladder.
  - Non-visualization of the gallbladder may occur in some normal subjects, from a stone in the cystic duct or subsequent fibrosis.

Hydrogen breath tests

  - **Lactulose breath test for bacterial overgrowth.** Oral lactulose is given, and excess gut flora in the small bowel or blind loop causes prompt metabolism to provide exhaled hydrogen.
  - **Lactose breath test for lactase deficiency.**
    - Oral lactose with subnormal exhaled hydrogen.

Renal investigations

Urine testing

Testing the urine is part of the routine physical examination. It is most simply done using one of the combination dipsticks.

- Dip the stick in the urine and compare the colours with the key at the times specified. Of particular interest are:
  - pH
  - protein content (**N.B.** does not detect Bence Jones protein)
  - ketones
  - glucose
  - bilirubin
  - urobilinogen
  - blood/haemoglobin

Urine microscopy

Urine should be sent to the laboratory (sterile) for 'M, C and S':

- M (microscopy)—for the presence of red cells, white cells, casts and pathogens.
- C (culture)—using appropriate media to detect bacteria and other pathogens.
- S (sensitivity)—to determine the sensitivity of bacteria to antibiotics.

Creatinine clearance

Precise measurements of the **glomerular filtration rate** are made isotopically, e.g. chromium EDTA clearance. The creatinine clearance is easier to organize, although less accurate.

- Collect a blood sample for plasma creatinine.
- Collect a 24-hour urine sample for creatinine.

$$\text{Formula: } \frac{U \times V}{P \times T}:$$

$$\frac{\text{Urine creatinine (mmol)}}{\text{Plasma creatinine } (\mu\text{mol})} \times \frac{\text{Urine volume (ml)} \times 10^3}{\text{Duration collection (min)}} = \text{Clearance (ml/min)}.$$

Normal value: 80–120 ml/min.

Intravenous urogram

An initial plain film to show renal or ureteric stones. Contrast medium is injected intravenously, concentrated in the kidney and excreted.

- Nephrogram phase—kidneys are outlined
    - observe position, size, shape, filling defects, e.g. tumour
- Excretion phase—renal pelvis
    - renal papillae may be lost from chronic pyelonephritis, papillary necrosis
    - calyces blunted from hydronephrosis
    - pelviureteric obstruction—large pelvis, normal ureters
- Ureters—observe position—displaced by other pathology?
    - size—dilated from obstruction or recent infection
    - irregularities—may be contractions and need to be checked in sequential films

Neurological investigations

Electroencephalogram

Approximately 22 electrodes are applied to the scalp in standard positions and cerebral electrical activity is amplified and recorded. There are marked normal variations and differences between awake and sleep.

Main uses

- Epilepsy
    - primary, generalized epilepsy—generalized spike and slow-wave discharges
    - partial epilepsy—focal spikes
- Disorders of consciousness or coma
    - encephalopathy
    - encephalitis
    - dementia

The main value of this technique is in showing episodes of abnormal waves compatible with epilepsy. Large normal variation makes interpretation difficult.

Lumbar puncture

A needle is introduced between the lumbar vertebrae (Fig. 11.17), through the dura into the subarachnoid space, and cerebrospinal fluid is obtained for examination.

Normal cerebrospinal fluid is completely clear.

The major diagnostic value of this technique is in:

- subarachnoid haemorrhage—uniformly red, whereas blood from a 'traumatic' tap is in the first specimen
  - xanthochromia—yellow stain from haemoglobin breakdown
- meningitis—pyogenic, turbid fluid, white cells, organisms on culture, low glucose and raised protein
- raised pressure may indicate a tumour

Myelogram

Inject contrast medium into cerebrospinal fluid in subarachnoid space to demonstrate thoracic or cervical disc prolapses or cord tumours.

Lumbar radiculogram

Inject contrast medium to demonstrate lumbar disc prolapses.

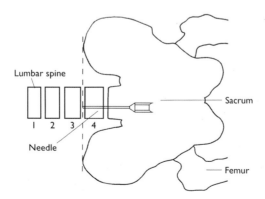

Fig. 11.17 The lumbar puncture needle is positioned between L3 and L4 to one side of the supraspinous ligament.

Haematological investigations

Full blood count and film examination

Blood should be taken into EDTA anticoagulant (purple top vacutainer) from venous puncture for analysis by automated cell counters. Most laboratories will be able to deliver the following parameters:

Hb (g/l or g/dl)	concentration of haemoglobin and the indicator of anaemia
RBC	red cell count, expressed as a number per litre
MCV (fl)	the mean cell volume; is useful in determining the cause of anaemia—microcytic (<76 fl), normocytic or macrocytic (>96 fl)
MCH (pg)	mean corpuscular haemoglobin measured in picograms; this defines hypochromia when <27 pg
MCHC	mean corpuscular haemoglobin concentration; not generally useful
WBC	total white cell count expressed as a number $\times 10^9$/l
Platelets	total platelet count expressed as a number $\times 10^9$/l

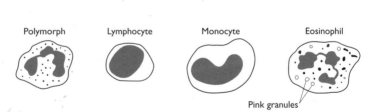

Polymorph   Lymphocyte   Monocyte   Eosinophil

Pink granules

Most automated blood analysers will provide a five part differential white cell count, thereby defining by percentage and absolute number of neutrophils, lymphocytes, monocytes, eosinophils and basophils present.

Blood film examination provides additional morphological information of blood cells and should always be requested in anaemia of unknown cause, abnormalities of white cell or platelet counts.

Red cells

Anaemia results from a reduction in the haemoglobin concentration—the causes of which include:

- bleeding
- haemolysis (premature destruction of red cells) — high reticulocyte count
- bone marrow disease (failure of production)
- haematinic deficiency (B_{12}, folate, iron)
- renal failure (reduction of erythropoietin)
- chronic inflammation and malignancy

The **MCV** is an indicator of the cause of anaemia:

- **Microcytic** — Fe deficiency, thalassaemia trait.
- **Macrocytic** — B_{12} or folate deficiency, hypothyroidism, liver disease, alcohol abuse and bone marrow disease.
- **Normochromic** — chronic disease, renal failure and malignancy.

Inspection of the **blood film** can provide useful information regarding the aetiology of anaemia. Red cell morphology is important in identifying causes of haemolysis, e.g. spherocytes, fragmented cells, sickle cells.

Haemoglobin electrophoresis. Electrophoresis of a red cell lysate will identify haemoglobin variants such as haemoglobin S-HbS. The detection and measurement of HbA_2 is very important for the detection of carriers of thalassaemia. HbA_2 >3.5% is suggestive of β-thalassaemia trait carrier status.

Red cell enzymes. Deficiency of red cell enzymes such as G6PD and PK can lead to a severe haemolytic anaemia. Such enzymes can be assayed in the laboratory.

White cells

An abnormal white cell count needs attention. Blood film examination may identify the presence of abnormal cells such as blasts, or, may simply show an elevation or reduction of normal components. The presence of abnormal white cell morphology may be an indication for a bone marrow biopsy.

- **Neutrophilia** — elevated neutrophil count; usually indicative of bacterial infection.
- **Neutropenia** — a low neutrophil count can lead to serious infection (gram-negative sepsis) often related to chemotherapy but temporarily may follow simple viral infection.

- **Lymphocytosis**—reactive in viral infections such as glandular fever; clonal in lymphoid leukaemias and lymphoma.
- **Lymphopenia**—common in patients taking steroids, human immunodeficiency virus (HIV), systemic lupus erythematosus (SLE) and other autoimmune disease.
- **Eosinophilia**—common in atopy and allergic states. Occurs in association with drugs, parasitic infection and lymphoma.

Coagulation

Blood should be taken into citrate (light blue-topped vacutainer tube). Citrate reversibly binds Ca^{2+} and prevents the sample from clotting. In the laboratory the blood is centrifuged and the plasma removed for testing. A source of tissue factor/phospholipid (thromboplastin) is added and Ca^{2+} added. The time to clot in seconds is measured.

o **Prothrombin time (PT)** (normally 10–14 seconds) is a measure of the extrinsic (tissue factor/VII dependent) system. It is very sensitive to vitamin K-dependent factors (II, VII, IX and X).
  - The PT is the most sensitive **liver function test**—prolonged in liver disease.
  - The PT is the most sensitive clotting test with which to **monitor warfarin therapy**—warfarin inhibits vitamin K-dependent clotting factors (II, VII, IX and X). The PT of the patient/PT of pooled normal plasma gives a ratio—the prothrombin ratio. If the PT ratio is multiplied by a correction for the 'sensitivity' of the thromboplastin used (international sensitivity ratio, ISI) the **INR** or **international normalized ratio** is derived.

Target INR	Clinical condition
2.0–3.0	Treatment of deep venous thrombosis (DVT) or pulmonary embolism (PE), anticoagulation in
3.0–4.5	recurrent DVT or PE, anticoaguation for prosthetic valves and grafts

o Activated partial thromboplastin time (APTT)—this measures the so-called intrinsic system. This pathway is slower and requires both phospholipid and a surface activator (e.g. kaolin—as in the kaolin cephalin thromboplastin time, KCTT). Patients' plasma from citrated blood is added to a source of phospholipid, kaolin and Ca^{2+}. The time to clot is measured and is usually in the order of 30–40 seconds). The test is used for:

— Monitoring heparin when the APTT is usually kept at about 2.5 × normal. **N.B.** low molecular weight heparin usually does not require monitoring with the exception of renal failure when a factor Xa assay is performed.
— This test is prolonged in the presence of the antiphospholipid antibody.
— The test is prolonged in haemophilia and von Willebrand's disease.

o **Other coagulation tests include the thrombin time (TT)** which is sensitive to heparin therapy and the **fibrinogen level** which is a direct measurement of the fibrinogen concentration of the blood. Disseminated intravascular coagulation usually causes a prolongation of all the above coagulation tests and a reduction in the level of fibrinogen.

o **D-dimers**—activation of the fibrinolytic system follows the formation of a clot. Plasmin becomes activated and cleaves the polymerized fibrin into smaller molecules (some of which are called D-dimers). D-dimers can be detected using either a latex agglutination or an ELISA-based test. The detection of D-dimers infers the presence of clot and is now used in the diagnosis of DVT and PE. Absence of D-dimers implies absence of significant thrombosis.

o **Thrombophilia tests**—a number of components of the blood help prevent the formation of spontaneous blood clots. These factors work by interupting the coagulation cascade. Deficiencies can make patients suseptible to thrombosis. Most of these factor deficiencies are inherited—**taking a family history is very important**. Main risk factors for thrombosis are:

— protein C deficiency
— protein S deficiency
— antithrombin III deficiency
— presence of a lupus anticoagulant (antiphospholipid antibody)
— oestrogen therapy—the pill
— surgery
— malignancy

Cross-matching blood for transfusion

Before blood can be safely administered to a patient, the patient's serum must be screened for red cell antibodies that may cause a transfusion rection should the corresponding antigen be present on the donor red cells. A sample of blood (varies in different laboratories—clot or EDTA) must be sent to the transfusion laboratory before blood can be issued. Careful labelling/identification of all samples is essential. Check with the transfusion laboratory as to what samples need to be taken and the system of labelling. The laboratory process involves.

- ABO and RhD blood grouping
- serum/plasma from patient is reacted with donor red cells
- once the ABO and RhD blood group has been determined and the absence of red cell antibodies has been confirmed, blood can be issued

Emergency blood for transfusion

There are rare occasions when there is insufficient time to allow for cross-matching. In this situation group O Rh-neg emergency stock can be given. (Must liase directly with transfusion laboratory.)

With the advent of highly sensitive red cell antibody screening techniques, routine cross-matching has been superseded by the electronic issue of ABO Rhesus compatible donor red cells for patients having a recent negative antibody screen. (This is not standard practice in all transfusion laboratories; refer to local transfusion policy.)

Special requirements

Certain patients have special transfusion requirements—some of these are listed here:

- **irradiated blood product**—patients will carry a card
- **cytomegalovirus (CMV)—negative blood products** may be required in:
  - patients undergoing organ transplantation
  - neonates

N.B. all blood issued in the UK is leucocyte depleted.

Bone marrow biopsy

This procedure is usually performed from the iliac crest (most often posterior) and is performed in two parts.

- The aspirate is marrow that is sucked out of the marrow cavity and spread on a glass slide, stained and examined under a microscope to determine cellular morphology. Staining of the marrow with Perl's Prussian blue stain will give the best indication as to the patient's iron status.
- The trephine involves taking a bone marrow core which is fixed in formalin, decalcified and then sectioned in the normal histological manner. The trephine will identify bone marrow infiltration with secondary carcinoma, fibrosis, haematological malignancies and best defines the cellularity of the marrow.

The procedure is either carried out with simple infiltration of the periosteum using local anaesthetic or under light sedation.

Bone marrow examination may give the following information:

- cellularity—i.e. whether the marrow is empty (aplastic anaemia), packed (leukaemia) or normal
- cytology—whether the cells within the marrow are maturing correctly and whether there are abnormal forms present
- iron status—the 'gold standard' against which other measurements of iron stores are tested

Biochemical tests

- **Urea and electrolytes**—measurement of sodium, potassium, urea and creatinine. Urea is useful in assessment of dehydration. It is dependant on protein loads—elevated by high protein meals or gastrointestinal bleeds, reduced by liver dysfunction. **Creatinine** is the most reliable test of glomerular function.
- **Anion gap**—difference in the sum of principal cations (sodium and potassium) and anions (chloride and bicarbonate) = 14–18 mmol/l (represents unmeasured negative charge on plasma proteins). Useful in investigation of acid–base alterations.
- **Liver functions tests**—better described as **liver profile** as the tests do not really reflect liver function.

- **Albumin**—mainly responsible for maintaining colloid osmotic pressure and a useful marker of liver synthetic function. May be dramatically reduced in nephrotic syndrome and protein-losing enteropathy.
- **AST and ALT** (aspartate transaminase and alanine amino transferase)—these enzymes are released in liver damage, but also present in red cells, muscle and cardiac cells. May be very high in hepatitis.
- **Bilirubin**—breakdown product of haemoglobin and therefore elevated in haemolysis. Also elevated in liver disease.
- **ALP** (alkaline phosphatase)—an enzyme found in osteoblasts and the hepatobiliary system. Elevated in bone disease and biliary obstruction.
- **GGT** (gamma glutamyl-transferase)—increased in alcohol abuse.
- **Amylase** enzyme produced by the pancreas for digestion of complex carbohydrates. Elevated in pancreatitis.

○ **Cardiac/muscle markers**
- **AST**—intrahepatic enzyme also found in skeletal and cardiac muscle. Elevated early in myocardial infarction (MI) but not specific.
- **LDH**—lactate dehydrogenase is found in many tissues. Rises more slowly in myocardial infarction (MI) and can be useful in retrospective diagnosis of MI.
- **CK-MB**—Creatine kinase isoenzyme found in cardiac muscle. More specific than AST and LDH but not infallible.
- **Troponins (T and I)**—most specific and sensitive markers of myocardial damage, rising early after myocardial injury. A rise in troponin is an indicator or risk in unstable angina and may indicate benefit from more aggressive treatment.

○ **Calcium/bone metabolism**
Most abundant mineral in the body, though 99% is bound within bone. Plasma levels need adjusting for the albumin concentration before interpretation.

Adjusted calcium = (40 − (albumin concentration (g/l)) × 0.02 mmol/l

Homeostasis of calcium is affected by parathyroid hormone (PTH) (↑) and vitamin D action.

- **Phosphate**—most commonly elevated in renal insufficiency. Very high levels are found in tumour lysis. Plasma levels affected by PTH and vitamin D action.
- **PTH**—released from parathyroid glands in response to a reduction in calcium and results in increased renal tubular absorption of calcium and increased phosphate excretion. Also releases calcium and phosphate from bone and leads to renal activation of vitamin D.
- **Vitamin D**—activated by hydroxylation in liver and kidney. Stimulates increased absorption of calcium and phosphate from the gut. Increases osteoblast bone resorption.

○ **Lipid profile (take samples fasting)**
- **Cholesterol**—important membrane structural component. Precursor of all steroid and bile acid synthesis. Elevated levels correlated with increased risk of cardiovacular disease, especially if LDL is elevated.
- **LDL (low density lipoprotein)**—principle carrier of cholesterol, attaching to LDL cell surface receptors to allow internalization. Independent cardiovascular risk factor.
- **HDL (high density lipoprotein)**—functions to reverse cholesterol transport, carrying cholesterol back to the liver for metabolism, therefore, cardioprotective.
- **Triglycerides**—present in dietary fat and synthesized by liver to provide store of energy. Independent cardiovascular risk factor. Elevated in liver disease and hypothyroidism.

Endocrinology

Anterior pituitary hormones

○ **TSH (thyroid stimulating hormone)**—stimulates production of thyroixine (T4) and tri-iodothyronine (T3) from the thyroid gland. Diagnosis of hypo- or hyperthyroidism depends on TSH measurement.
○ **ACTH (adrenocorticotrophic hormone)**—increases cortisol production from the adrenal glands in response to stress, daily variation, infection, etc.
- Cortisol excess is known as Cushing's syndrome or Cushing's disease (pituitary-driven ACTH).

- Cortisol deficiency from adrenal failure is known as Addison's disease.

o **GH (growth hormone)**—stimulates growth in prepubertal children and has many diffuse effects on adult metabolism. GH is activated by insulin-like growth factor 1 (IGF-1) in the liver. An excess of growth hormone in adulthood produces acromegaly.

o **Prolactin**—milk gland stimulating hormone elevated in pregnancy and lactation. Very high levels in some pituitary adenomata.

o **FSH (follicle stimulating hormone)**—gonadotrophin which nurtures the development of the follicle in the first half of the menstraul cycle. In males FSH stimulates spermatogenesis. High levels are found in post-menopausal women.

o **LH (luteinizing hormone)**—elevated in the second half of the menstrual cycle producing development of the corpus luteum. In males LH stimulates testosterone synthesis.

Posterior pituitary hormone

o **ADH (antidireutic hormone)**—decreases water loss. Absence of ADH causes diabetes insipidus. Conditions that cause inappropriate ADH secretion (various tumours) lead to a fall in plasma sodium. Measurement of **urine and plasma osmolarity.**

Dynamic endocrine tests

o **Short Synacthen test**—injection of synthetic ACTH at time 0 after blood sampling. Further blood samples are taken at 30 and 60 minutes. A physiological response results in an elevation of cortisol peak to >570 nmol/l. A reduced response is seen in Addison's disease (adrenal failure).

o **Oral glucose tolerance test (OGTT)**—used to diagnose diabetes mellitus by demonstrating abnormal glucose handling.

o **Insulin tolerance test**—used to demonstrate the normal reactivity of cortisol and growth hormone (both antagonize the action of insulin) to hypoglycaemia induced by insulin. Abnormal response seen in adrenal failure or growth hormone deficiency.

o **Testing for Cushing's syndrome**
   - **Outpatient screening test**

Table 11.1 Diagnosis of glycaemic status.

Diagnosis	Timing	Plasma glucose (mmol/l)
Physiological	Fasting	<6.1
Impaired fasting	Fasting	>6.1 <7.0
glucose	2-hour OGTT	<7.8
Impaired glucose	Fasting	<7.0
tolerance	2-hour OGTT	>7.8 <11.1
Diabetes mellitus	Fasting	>7.0
	2-hour OGTT	>11.1

- **1 mg overnight dexamethasone suppression test** — 1 mg of dexamethasone is administered at 11.00 pm or midnight; clotted or lithium heparin sample for cortisol measurement is taken at 8.00–9.00 am (supraphysiological steroid dose should suppress endogenous production when cortisol is sampled next morning).
- **Urinary cortisol output** — 24-hour urine collection to measure urinary free cortisol.
- **Inpatient screening tests — liase with endocrinologists.** Involves low and high dose dexamethasone suppression tests, midnight cortisol sampling and radiological examination of the pituitary, adrenals and any other relevant ectopic source.

Immunological investigations

o **Antinuclear antibody** — Can be of any immunoglobulin (Ig) class. Staining pattern is associated with specific diseases:

Homogeneous	lupus
Speckled	mixed connective tissue disease
Nucleolar staining	scleroderma
Centromere staining	CREST syndrome (calcinosis, Raynaud's phenomenon, oesophageal motility abnormalities, scleroderma and telangiectasia)

o **Antismooth muscle antibody** — elevated in autoimmune hepatitis.

- **Gastric parietal cell**—seen in patients with pernicious anaemia (90%).
- **Intrinsic factor antibodies**—70% of pernicious anaemia patients; more specific.
- **Mitochondrial antibody**—96% of patients with primary biliary cirrhosis.
- **Anti-endomysial and antigliadin antibodies**—coeliac disease.
- **Thyroid antibody**—antithyroglobulin elevated in autoimmune thyroiditis (90%); antimicrosomal antibody elevations may be seen in Grave's disease.
- **Rheumatoid factor**—antibody against human IgG but can be of any Ig class. Positive in 70% of rheumatoid arthritis, particularly extra-articular involvement. Very high levels in cryoglobulinaemia.
- **ANCA (antineutrophil cytoplasmic antibodies)**
  - **Cytoplasmic ANCA (cANCA)**—90% of Wegener's granulomatosis; 40% of patients with microscopic polyangiitis.
  - **Perinuclear ANCA (pANCA)**—60% of microscopic polyangiitis patients; may also be positive in connective tissue disorders and vasculitic diseases.

Taking blood samples

Venepuncture

Wear plastic gloves when taking blood. Venous blood is normally taken from a vein in the antecubital fossa—it is not necessary to clean the area with a swab, unless dirt is apparent. **DO NOT TAKE BLOOD FROM AN ARM WITH A DRIP.**

- Place a tourniquet above the elbow or inflate a cuff to approximately 50–80 mmHg.
- Ask patient to make a clenched fist repeatedly.
- Inspect for superficial vein. If not seen, palpate with fingertip repeatedly across antecubital fossa for rebound from a tense vein. Map out course of vein.
- Make sure the vessel is not pulsating (i.e. is the brachial artery).
- Decide where you wish to insert needle—a site over the middle of the vein, along line of vein.

- Place your thumb on skin firmly below the proposed puncture site and move towards you to stretch skin.
- Insert needle firmly through the skin at an angle of about 20°.

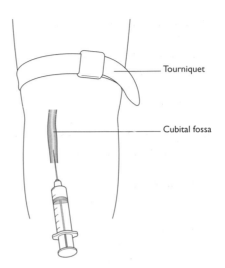

Tourniquet

Cubital fossa

Syringe/needle

Place a relatively wide-bore needle on appropriate-sized syringe.

- Place needle on the skin over middle of vein, and insert needle, as above.
- As soon as the needle appears to be in the vein, pull the syringe plunger back slowly until you have the amount of blood required.
- It is common to go through vein—if after inserting needle no blood appears, withdraw syringe/needle gently with sustained pull on the plunger: sudden ingress of blood into syringe denotes success.
- If no success, before needle is removed from skin, push again along a different line and withdraw as above.
- Release the tourniquet, before taking the needle out, or blood will leak out of the puncture site profusely.
- Place your thumb over a piece of cotton-wool on the puncture site and press when you have withdrawn needle.
- Ask the patient to maintain pressure for about 2 minutes.
- A small plaster on site protects patient's clothing from any leak.
- If a bleed occurs, maintain pressure for longer and elevate the arm to assist clotting by reducing venous pressure.

Becton–Dickinson vacutainer system

Insert the end of the needle with a covering rubber sleeve into a plastic holder.

- Carry out venepuncture, as above, holding the plastic holder to insert needle.
- When you think you are in the vein, push appropriate tube into the plastic holder, where its rubber bung is pierced by the proximal end of the needle. The vacuum in the tube automatically withdraws the blood. Repeated tubes can be filled in the same way without withdrawing the needle from the vein.

Blood sample bottles (vacutainers):

> Purple (EDTA) — full blood count.
> Blue (citrate reversibly chelates calcium) — coagulation tests.
> Green (heparin) — biochemistry.
> Grey (contains fluoride to inhibit glycolysis) for measurement of blood glucose.
> Brown (no anticoagulatant) — for tests on serum such as immunology, microbiology serology.

Blood cultures

Remember to swab the tops of bottles before piercing the seal with needle. Change needle between skin and bottle.

For both methods

- Dispose of the needle and syringe carefully.
- Do not use a tourniquet for calcium samples.
- If you cannot obtain blood from the antecubital fossa, try 'houseman's' vein over lateral surface of radius at wrist, or vein in forearm or on the back of the hand.

Arterial blood-gas estimation

This is not an easy procedure. Watch it being done before you attempt it yourself.

Use a 2-ml syringe and draw up a small quantity of heparin. Expel the heparin so just a film remains in the syringe. Pre-prepared syringes are now available. In nervous patients, infiltrate the skin with lignocaine to decrease discomfort.

— **Radial artery.** Make sure the arm is in a stable horizontal position. Palpate the middle of the artery. Insert the needle into the artery at 45°. Gradually withdraw the needle until blood flows freely into the syringe. Fill the sy-

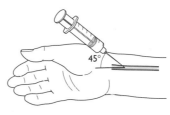

ringe with blood and remove it with the needle attached. Press firmly on the puncture site and ask the patient to press for a further 5 minutes. Remove the needle and put an air-tight cap over the syringe nozzle. Make sure sample is analysed within 5–10 minutes.

— **Femoral artery.** Make sure the patient is lying flat. Palpate the artery and insert the needle at 90°. Remember the femoral nerve lies laterally to the femoral artery and the femoral vein medially. Proceed as above.

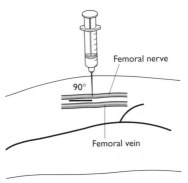

— Points to remember:
  — avoid air bubbles in the sample
  — note oxygen concentration the patient is breathing (air, 24%, 28%, etc.)
  — in nervous patients you made need to infiltrate the skin with lignocaine
  — arterial blood is bright red. It is easy to hit the femoral vein which provides dark red blood. The radial artery is preferred for this reason

Hyper- and hypoglycaemia

Blood glucose

Colorimetric methods

Several proprietary glucose-oxidase colour strips are available. Examples include strips for use with meters, or visual use. Make sure the strips have been kept in a sealed container.

- Prick finger with a lancet, and squeeze fingertip to produce drop of blood.
- Put one large drop of blood on to the pad on the strip or meter's detector—a smear will **not** do.
- Follow instructions for visual reading, maybe to time precisely for 1 minute (use second hand of watch or digital watch).
  - Some methods require you to wipe off blood using cotton wool or tissue paper; wait 1 more minute before reading strip.
- Use a colorimeter for a more precise reading, particularly in the hypoglycaemic range.

Amperometric methods

Some machines give a direct current output from a glucose-oxidase strip.
  - After applying blood to the strip, the result is shown after about 20 seconds.

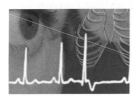

CHAPTER 12

The 12-Lead Electrocardiogram

Introduction

The electrocardiogram (ECG) tracings arise from the electrical changes, depolarization and repolarization that accompany muscle contraction. With knowledge of the relative position of the leads to the electrodes, the ECG tracings provide direct information of the cardiac muscle and its activity.

Six **standard leads**—I, II, III, aVR, aVL, aVF—are recorded from the

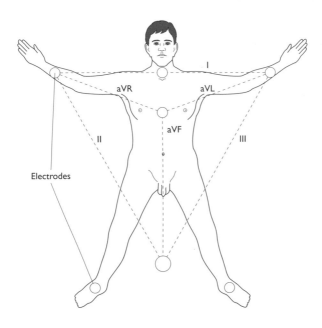

Electrodes

limb electrodes (aV = augmented voltage) and examine the heart from different directions.

The standard leads examine the heart in the **vertical** plane.

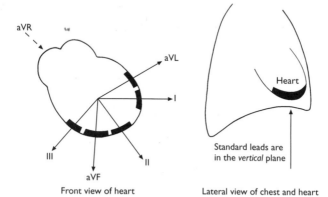

Front view of heart

Lateral view of chest and heart

Standard leads are in the *vertical* plane

Six chest leads, V leads, attached by sticky electrodes to the chest wall, are all in the **horizontal** plane.

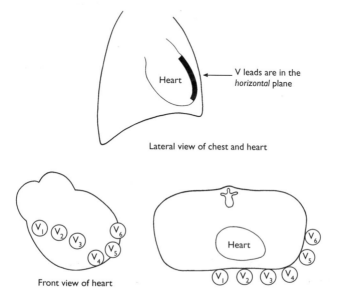

Lateral view of chest and heart

V leads are in the *horizontal* plane

Front view of heart

Obstruction of arteries gives appropriate specific patterns of ischaemia:

— left anterior descending coronary artery—*anterior ischaemia* or *infarct* (V_{1-6})
— circumflex coronary artery—*lateral ischaemia* or *infarct* (I, aVL)
— right coronary artery—*inferior ischaemia* or *infarct* (II, III, aVF)

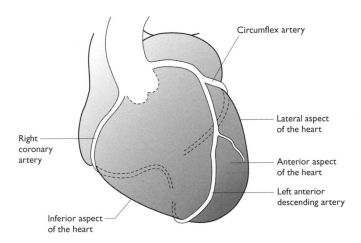

Every ECG tracing must first be standardized by making sure the 1 mV mark deviates the pointer 10 small squares on the paper.

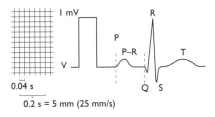

P = atrial depolarization, QRS = ventricular depolarization, T = repolarization.

Normal ECG

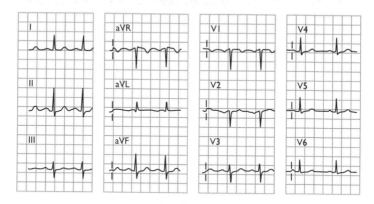

Fig. 12.1 A normal electrocardiogram.

Normal ECG variants

- T waves can be inverted in leads III, aVF, V$_{1-3}$.
- T waves and P waves are always inverted in aVR (if not, leads are misplaced).
- In a young athletic person:
  - ST segments may be raised, especially in leads V$_{1-5}$
  - right bundle-branch block (RBBB) may occur
  - electrical criteria of left ventricular hypertrophy may be present
  - bradycardia <40 beats/min
  - physiological Q waves
- Ectopics of any type, including ventricular, are rarely of significance.
- Raised ST segments are common in Afro-Caribbean subjects.
- P mitrale is overdiagnosed:
  - P wave in V$_1$ is often biphasic

Electrophysiology of cardiac contractions

All cardiac muscle has a tendency to depolarization, leading to excitation and contraction.

Initial electrical discharge from sinoatrial (SA) node (under influence of sympathetic and parasympathetic control) spreads to atrioventricular (AV) node and via bundle of His to ventricles.

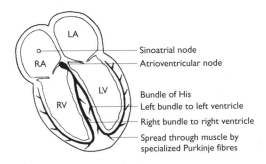

The deflection of the ECG tracing indicates the average direction of all muscle activity at each moment.

Depolarization spreads:
- towards lead—ECG tracing moves up the paper
- away from lead—tracing moves down paper

P wave

- depolarization spreads from SA node to AV node through the atrial muscle fibres (1 in figure below)
- best seen in leads II and V₁
- usually small, as atria are small

Normal P wave <2.5 mm high, <2.5 mm wide

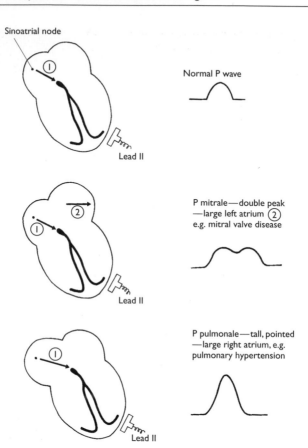

Sinoatrial node

Lead II

Normal P wave

P mitrale—double peak
—large left atrium ②
e.g. mitral valve disease

Lead II

P pulmonale—tall, pointed
—large right atrium, e.g.
pulmonary hypertension

Lead II

QRS complex

The QRS deflections have a standard nomenclature:

Q—any initial deflection downwards.

R—any deflection upwards, whether or not a preceding Q.

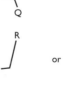 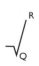

S—any deflection downwards after an R
wave, whether or not a preceding Q.

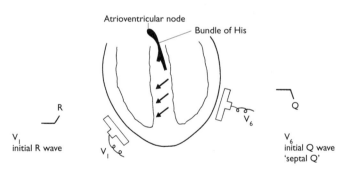

QRS in the V leads

Usually: V$_{1-2}$
opposite
R ventricle

V$_{3-4}$
opposite
septum

V$_{5-6}$
opposite
L ventricle

The septum depolarizes first from left to right.

V$_1$
initial R wave

V$_6$
initial Q wave
'septal Q'

The ventricles then depolarize from inside outwards. The large left
ventricle then normally dominates.

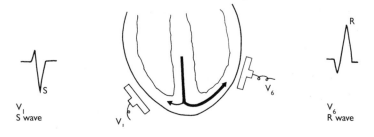

V$_1$
S wave

V$_6$
R wave

The transition point where R and S are equal is the position of the septum.

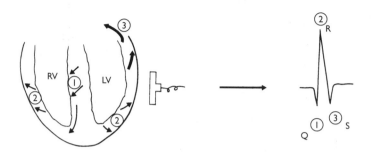

V_6 S wave after R wave as depolarization spreads around ventricle away from V_6.

Left-ventricle hypertrophy (LVH)

V_5 or V_6 — R wave >25mm.
V_1 or V_2 — S wave deep.
Tallest R wave + deepest S wave >35mm.

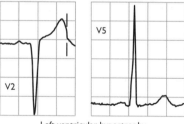

Left ventricular hypertrophy

- Voltage changes on their own are not enough — thin people with a thin ribcage can have big complexes.
- Obese people have small complexes.
- Also look for R wave in V_1 — rotation to right of transition point left axis deviation.
- T-wave inversion in V_5, V_6 in the presence of LVH is termed left ventricular 'strain pattern' and indicates marked hypertrophy.

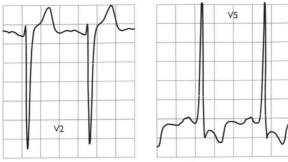

Left ventricular hypertrophy with strain

Right-ventricle hypertrophy (RVH)

The left ventricle is no longer dominant.

V_1 — R wave > S wave.

V_6 — deep S wave.

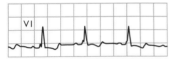
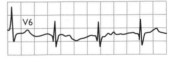

Right ventricular hypertrophy

— Also look for:
    — right axis deviation
    — peaked P of right atrial hypertrophy
    — T-wave inversion in V_2 and V_3 — right ventricular 'strain pattern'

Myocardial infarction (MI)—full thickness of ventricle

Infarction is the term for dead muscle.

Pathological Q wave:
    — width = or >0.04 seconds (one small square)
    — depth > one-third height of R wave
    — smaller Q waves are physiological from septum depolarization
    — as ventricles depolarize from inside, an electrode in the ventricle cavity would record contraction as Q wave

- through 'dead' window, this is seen as if from inside the heart, i.e. the depolarization of the far ventricle wall away from the electrode gives a negative deflection

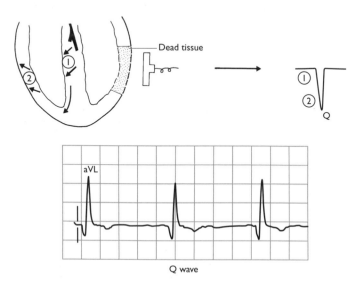

Q wave

Acute myocardial ischaemia—raised ST segments

Damaged but potentially salvagable myocardium:
- ST segment—normally within 0.5mm of isoelectric line
- ST elevation in V_1 and V_2 may be normal—high 'take -off' of j point
- ST elevation elsewhere is normal

Normal baseline:
Resting myocardial cell potential approximately −90mV. In an injured cell, failing cell membrane only allows potential of perhaps −40mV.

Resting potential in
normal myocardial cell

Resting potential in
injured myocardial cell

If two electrodes record from different areas of the resting heart, one normal and one injured, a galvanometer would register −50mV (i.e. the difference between −90mV and −40mV). This depresses the baseline below normal over the injured area, although this cannot be recognized until after QRS complex.

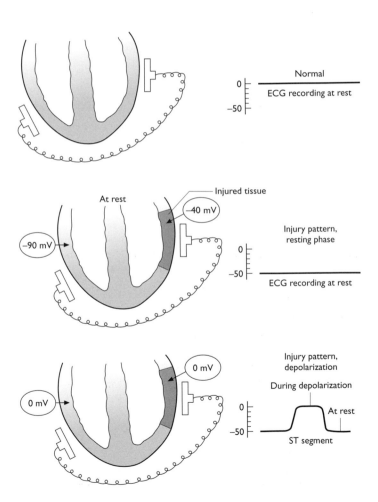

Normal

ECG recording at rest

Injury pattern, resting phase

ECG recording at rest

Injury pattern, depolarization

During depolarization

At rest

ST segment

Table 12.1 Classical time sequence of onset of ECG changes in myocardial infarction.

Approximate time of onset after chest pain			ECG changes
Immediately	1.	May be normal	ECG may be normal. Occasionally ST segment changes occur immediately pain develops, or even before
0–2 hours	2.		ST segments rise—occluded artery → injury pattern
3–8 hours	3.		Injured tissue remains Some dies (Q waves = myocardium death) Some improves to become ischaemic only (T-wave inversion) Full infarct pattern: – Q waves – raised ST segments – inverted T waves
8–24 hours	4.		Injured tissue either dies → Q wave or improves and abnormal ST segments disappear Inverted T waves remain
After 1–2 days	5.		Ischaemia disappears T waves upright again Q waves usually remain, as dead tissue will not not come alive again

Q waves may subsequently disappear if scarred tissue contracts.

Raised ST segment:
- acute ischaemic injury of ventricle
- pericarditis
- normal athletes
- normal West Indians

Anterior infarction (Figs 12.2 and 12.3)
- changes in leads V_{1-6}
    - occlusion of left anterior descending coronary artery

Inferior infarction (Fig. 12.4)
- changes in leads II, III, aVF
    - occlusion of right coronary artery

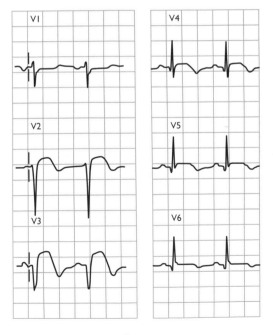

Fig. 12.2 Acute anterior infarct: ST ↑ V_{2-6} at 3–8 hours.

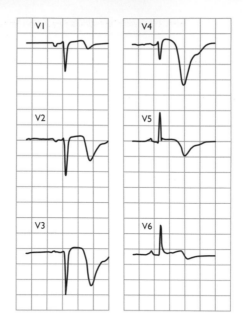

Fig. 12.3 Ten hours after anterior myocardial infarct.

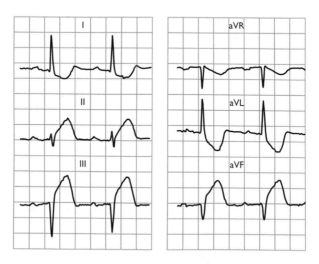

Fig. 12.4 Acute inferior infarct: ST ↑ in II, III, a VF with reciprocal depression in other leads.

Lateral infarction
- changes in leads I, aVL
    - occlusion of circumflex artery

Septal infarction
- changes in leads V_{2-3}
    - occlusion of septal branches of left anterior descending coronary artery

Posterior infarction
- changes in lead V_1 (e.g. R wave, ST depression)
    - occlusion of branches of right coronary artery

Chronic myocardial ischaemia
Reduced oxygen supply to muscle:
- ST depression
- T-wave inversion
- occasionally tall pointed T wave

These changes can also occur during an exercise tolerance test when ischaemia develops:

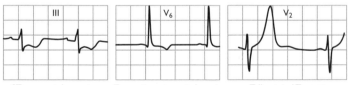

ST segment depression   T-wave inversion—ischaemic   Tall pointed T waves

QRS axis
- The direction of depolarization of the heart is sometimes helpful in diagnosis.
- Note the axis deviation on its own is rarely significant but alerts you to look for right or left ventricular hypertrophy.
- Look at the standard leads for the most equiphasic QRS complex (R and S equal). The axis is approximately at right angles to this in the direction of the most positive standard lead (largest R wave).

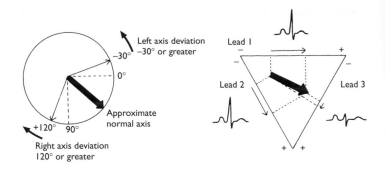

Pattern recognition

Left axis deviation

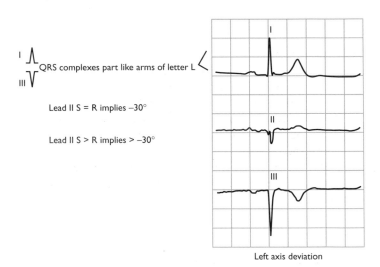

I ⋀
⎻⎺⊤⎺ QRS complexes part like arms of letter L
III ⋁

Lead II S = R implies −30°

Lead II S > R implies > −30°

Left axis deviation

Right axis deviation

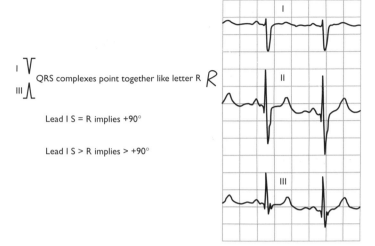

I ⋁

III ⋏   QRS complexes point together like letter R   R

Lead I S = R implies +90°

Lead I S > R implies > +90°

QRS complex

- Normal if width <0.12 second (three small squares).
- If >0.12 second—bundle-branch block.
- An apparently wide QRS complex, <0.12 second wide—partial bundle-branch block or interventricular conduction defect.
- Left bundle-branch block (LBBB) is usually associated with some form of heart disease.
- RBBB is often a normal variation, especially in athletes. Immediately after a myocardial infarction the development of RBBB may be serious.

Left bundle-branch block

- M pattern in V_6.
- Throughout ECG, slurred ST segment and T wave inversion opposite to major deflection of QRS.
- Lead V_6
  - depolarization of septal muscle from right bundle gives positive deflection

- right heart depolarization gives negative deflection
- left heart depolarization gives positive deflection

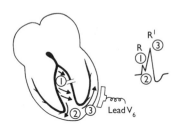

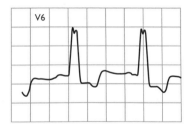

- Standard leads
- left axis deviation as impulse spreads from right bundle up to left ventricle
- also occurs if only anterior fascicle of left bundle blocked
    - left anterior hemiblock

Right bundle-branch block
- M pattern in V_1.
- Lead V_1
- depolarization of septal muscle from left bundle gives positive deflection
- left heart depolarization gives negative deflection
- right heart depolarization gives positive deflection

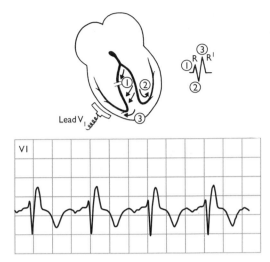

- Standard leads
  - axis usually normal, as depends on large muscle mass of left ventricle
  - if RBBB is associated with left axis, there is block of anterior fascicle of left bundle—bifascicular block

    All heart is being excited via remaining posterior fascicle of left bundle.

Arrhythmias
  - sinus arrhythmia
  - ectopics
  - tachycardias
  - bradycardias

Sinus arrhythmia
Normal variation with respiratory rate—increase rate on inspiration.

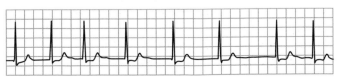

Ectopics

Atrial ectopics

Ectopic focus anywhere in atria. Depolarization spreads across atrium to AV node like any normal beat:

— P wave is abnormal shape

— normal QRS complex

The atrial ectopic focus must fire early — or would be entrained by normal excitation:

— appears early on rhythm strip

— followed by compensatory pause — waiting for normal SA node cycle

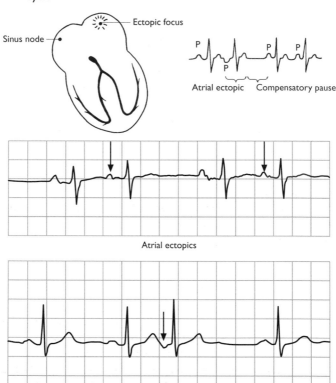

Atrial ectopics

Atrial ectopic — an inverted P wave

Junctional or nodal ectopics

Ectopic at AV node; no P wave.

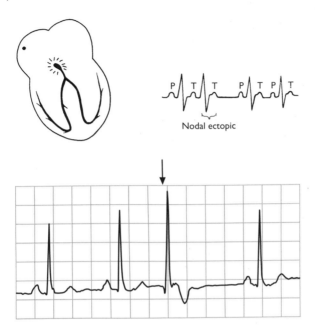

Nodal ectopic

Ventricular ectopics

Ectopic anywhere in ventricles. Depolarization occurs first in that ventricle then spreads to other ventricle:

- no P wave
- wide complex
- bundle branch-block pattern
  - left focus — RBBB pattern
  - right focus — LBBB pattern

Atrial and junctional ectopics are invariably innocent when picked up on a random ECG. The majority of ventricular ectopics are also innocent except after a myocardial infarction. Ventricular ectopics picked up on routine monitoring of healthy patients are approximately proportional to age, i.e. 30% of 30-year-olds, 50% of 50-year-olds and almost 100% of 70-year-olds. Innocent ventricular ectopics usually disappear on exercise.

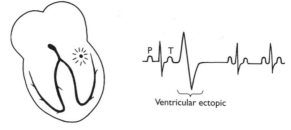

Ventricular ectopic

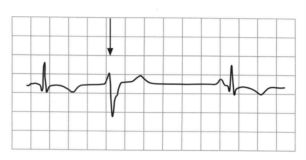

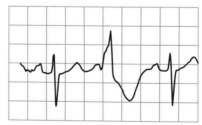

Tachycardias

Classification of tachycardias
- **O** Tachycardias are divided into:
    - **Narrow-complex regular** — QRS complex up to 0.08 seconds — two little squares on ECG
    - sinus tachycardia

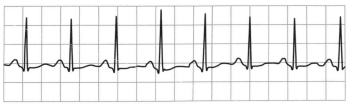

Sinus tachycardia

- supraventricular tachycardia, atrial tachycardia, atrial flutter
- **Narrow-complex irregular**
    - atrial tachycardia with varying block, atrial fibrillation
- **Broad-complex**—QRS complex about 0.12 seconds—three small squares
    - ventricular arrhythmias and occasionally supraventricular with aberrant (delayed) conduction
○ Deciding whether a tachycardia is **atrial** or **ventricular** is not easy. Here are some pointers.
    - Narrow-complex tachycardias are usually atrial and broad-complex usually ventricular, **but not always**.
    - When acute ischaemic heart disease is present, tachycardias are usually ventricular. In the absence of ischaemic heart disease tachycardias are usually atrial, **but not always**.
    - If there is independent atrial activity (random appearance of p values), the tachycardia is ventricular.
    - Look at the patient's preceding ECGs or rhythm strip. If the tachycardia looks like a previous ectopic beat in shape, it will be that type of tachycardia.
    - Vagal stimulation (rubbing carotid, etc.) will only be effective in atrial rhythms.
    - The regularity or irregularity is not helpful in distinguishing ventricular from atrial arrhythmias.

Atrial fibrillation
The electrical impulse and contraction travel randomly around the atria:
    - 'bag-of-worms' quivering atria
    - irregular little waves on ECG—best seen V₁

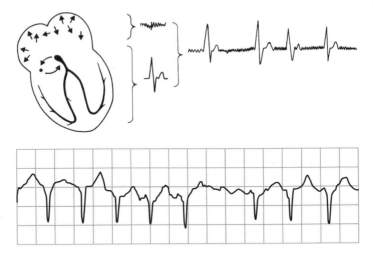

When it first develops, often 150+, fibrillation waves are difficult to see:

— AV node fires irregularly
— normal QRS complexes

   If irregular rate, no P waves, normal QRS — likely to be atrial fibrillation.

Digoxin is still the drug of choice — it decreases transmission of impulses down the bundle of His.

Atrial flutter

Atria contract very rapidly, 200–250 beats/min, giving a sawtooth pattern, but the ventricles only respond to every second or third or fourth contraction (2:1, 3:1, 4:1 block).

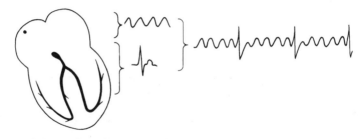

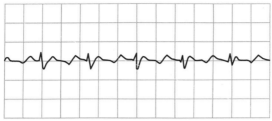

2 : 1 atrial flutter

Treated with digoxin, normally changes to atrial fibrillation.

Supraventricular tachycardia (SVT)

- Arises near AV node, 170 beats/min or more, regular.
- Complexes are identical, normal width or wide if also bundle-branch block.
- Common in young patients (20–30 years).
- Rarely represents heart disease.
- Sudden onset and finish.
- Last few minutes to several hours.
- May be tired, light-headed, uncomfortable.
- In older patients SVTs more likely to represent heart disease.

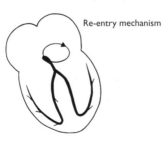

Re-entry mechanism

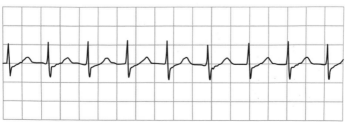

Vagal stimulation (rubbing carotid sinus) can terminate attack.

Re-entry is the most common mechanism for tachycardias (Fig. 12.5). Assumes two conduction pathways lead to ventricles. Normally conduction passes equally quickly down both pathways.

Problems arise when one pathway recovers more slowly than the other. When this happens the next conduction passes down only one pathway.

Conduction subsequently passes retrogradely up the other pathway, which is no longer refractory. This pathway then becomes refractory while the first pathway conducts again and the impulse races round the pathways to give a tachycardia.

Wolff–Parkinson–White syndrome

This is the classic re-entry arrhythmia. There are two separate pathways from the atria to the ventricles. In the resting ECG the early entry, by the aberrant conduction pathway bypassing the bundle of His, is seen as a delta wave.

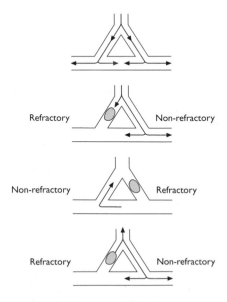

Fig. 12.5 The mechanism of re-entry tachycardias.

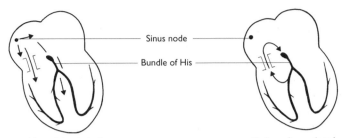

Normal depolarization
in the WPW syndrome

Tachycardia produced
via accessory pathway
in WPW syndrome

Sinus node

Bundle of His

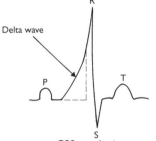

Delta wave

P

R

T

S

QRS complex in
WPW syndrome

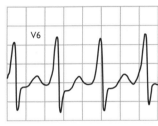

V6

Ventricular tachycardia

- Potentially dangerous rhythm which can develop into ventricular fibrillation.
- Rapid but not as fast as SVT (usually less than 170 beats/min).
- Often slightly irregular.
- Patient often looks collapsed.
- Always wide QRS complex
  - LBBB pattern—right focus
  - RBBB pattern—left focus

Treatment is with lignocaine 100mg intravenously at once with transfer of the patient to hospital.

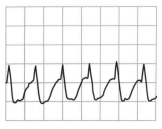

Re-entry mechanism

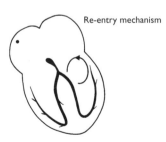

Bradycardias
Pulse rate <60 beats/min.

Sinus
Normal P wave and QRS complexes.

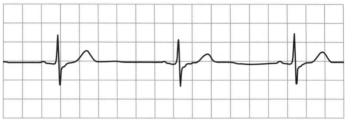

Sinus bradycardia

○ **Causes:**
- – athletic heart
- – β-blockers
- – hypothyroidism
- – raised intracranial pressure
- – pain with vagal response
  - – dental pain
  - – glaucoma
  - – biliary colic

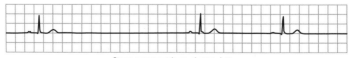

Sinus arrest with vagal stimulation

First-degree heart block

- PR interval (beginning of P wave to beginning of QRS complex) >0.22 second (5.5 little squares).
- Depolarization delayed in the region of AV node.

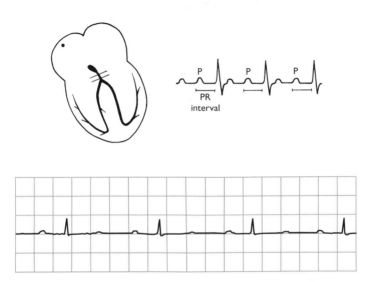

Wenckebach heart block

In a cycle of three or four beats the PR interval gradually lengthens until a P wave appears on its own with no QRS complex. The cycle then repeats itself.

Gradually increasing PR interval until a QRS is dropped

2:1 Block

The QRS complexes only respond to every other P wave, i.e. every other P wave has no QRS complex.

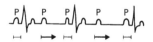

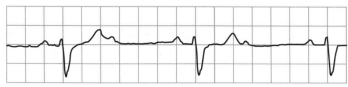

2 : 1 heart block

Complete heart block

- No relation between P waves and QRS complex.
- Inherent ventricular rate about 40 beats/min.
- QRS complex abnormal as it arises in a ventricular focus.

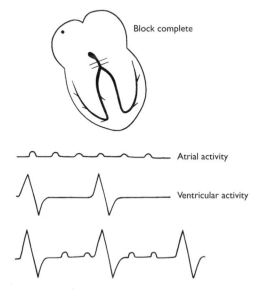

Block complete

Atrial activity

Ventricular activity

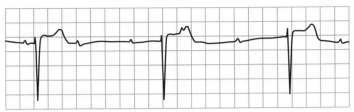

Complete heart block

Pacemakers

- When conduction defects cause asystolic pauses or very slow heart rates, pacemakers can stimulate either the atrium or ventricle and restore rhythm.
- Pacemakers can be basic or very sophisticated.

Ventricle-only pacemakers

These are the commonest types of pacemaker (80%+). If the ventricle fails to produce an electrical signal (QRS complex), the pacemaker senses this

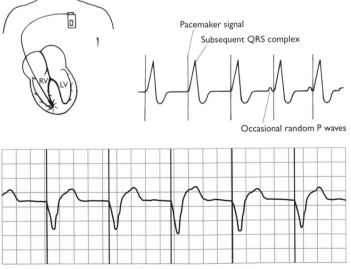

Pacemaker signal

Subsequent QRS complex

Occasional random P waves

Ventricular pacing

and fires at approximately 60–70 beats/min. It is inhibited when the ventricles QRS complex returns at an adequate rate.

Atrial-only pacemakers

In the sick sinus syndrome, the P wave fails to materialize but conduction in the AV node and bundle of His is normal. Pacing the atrium restores normal function.

Sequential pacemakers

These pacemakers cause the sequential contraction of the atrium and ventricle in a more normal physiological way. This may provide a better cardiac output.

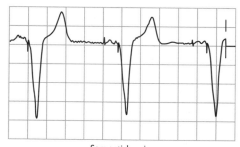

Sequential pacing

Looking at the ECG

Examine logically, reading complexes from left to right.
- **Rhythm:**
    - sinus rhythm ± ectopics. Ignore sinus arrhythmia
    - regular
        - slow complete heart block
        - sinus bradycardia
        - fast sinus tachycardia
        - supraventricular tachycardia
        - ventricular tachycardia
        - regular atrial flutter

- irregular
    - atrial fibrillation
    - atrial tachycardia with varying block
o **Rate:** add up the number of large squares between two successive beats. Divide into 300. For example:

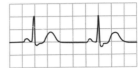

$$\frac{300}{5 \text{ large squares}} = 60 \text{ beats/min}$$

1.5 squares = 200 beats/min 3.5 = 85 beats/min

2	= 150 beats/min	4	= 75 beats/min
2.5	= 120 beats/min	5	= 60 beats/min
3	= 100 beats/min	6	= 50 beats/min

If the simple formula does not work for irregular rhythm—then add up number of complexes in 6 seconds (sometimes marked on the paper) and multiply by 10.

o **Complex shape**—brief guide:
    - P wave: abnormal shape
        - atrial ectopics, P mitrale, P pulmonale
        - 0.10–0.22 second (2.5–5.5 squares)
    - PR interval: prolonged
        - >0.22 second: first-degree heart block
        - <0.1 second: Wolff–Parkinson–White syndrome
    - QRS complex
        - large Q wave—full-thickness infarct?
        - wide QRS >0.12 second: branch block
        - R wave if large: ventricular hypertrophy?
    - ST segment: elevated or depressed—ischaemia or other causes?
    - T wave: if inverted—ischaemia or other causes?

In summary, particularly look for:
o abnormal rhythm
o abnormal rate
o abnormal QRS—especially ischaemia, infarct, hypertrophy

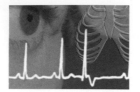

CHAPTER 13

Interpretation of Investigations

Sensitivity, specificity and efficiency

These terms have specific meanings which indicate the clinical usefulness of investigations. Sensitivity and specificity assess the frequency of results in relation to the correct answers.

		Correct diagnosis	
		+	−
Test result	+	true positive	false positive
	−	false negative	true negative

o **Sensitivity**—how often the correct positive answer is obtained in those who have the disease:

$$= \frac{\text{True-Positive}}{\text{True-positive} + \text{false-negative}}, \text{ i.e.}$$

It also expresses the likelihood that a negative test result correctly indicates disease is not present: 95% sensitivity means five false-negatives in 100 patients with the disease.

o **Specificity**—how often the correct negative answer is obtained in those who do not have the disease:

$$= \frac{\text{True-negative}}{\text{True-negative} + \text{false-positive}}, \text{ i.e.}$$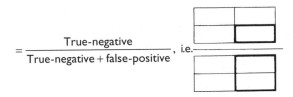

It also expresses the likelihood that a positive test result will correctly indicate disease: 90% specificity means 10 false-positives in 100 subjects tested who do not have the disease.

Thus a large heart on X-ray is a fairly sensitive test for severe mitral regurgitation (most patients with mitral regurgitation have a large heart) but it is not a specific test (because many heart diseases produce a large heart).

o **Efficiency**—how often the investigation gives the correct answer:

$$= \frac{\text{True-positive} + \text{true-negative}}{\text{All tests}}, \text{ i.e.}$$

o **Predictive value of a positive test**

$$= \frac{\text{True-positive}}{\text{True-positive} + \text{false-positive}}, \text{ i.e.}$$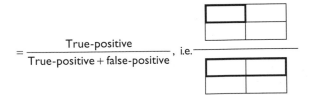

Interpretation

The reliance put on the result of an investigation depends on the *a priori* chance of the result being abnormal. Thus a high plasma calcium in a woman with breast cancer would be taken to indicate either bone metastases or the non-metatastic hypercalcaemia (due to tumour production of a parathormone-like peptide), whereas a similar value in an apparently normal medical student would be regarded as being a false-positive until rechecked. Where the prior probability of an event is known, Bayes theorem can be used to calcuate the current probability. The prevalence of an abnormality in the population therefore assists interpretation of an individual patient's results.

Prevalence and incidence

Please note the difference between prevalence and incidence.

- **Prevalence** — the number of cases of a disease in a designated population, e.g. 10% of males aged 40–60 years.
- **Incidence** — the number of new cases during a specific period, e.g. 10 per 100 000 population per annum.

CHAPTER 14

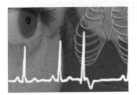

Laboratory Results —
Normal Values

Introduction

Normal ranges are the most frequently used reference interval. For some situations, **specific diagnostic reference intervals** are appropriate, e.g. twice normal value of plasma creatine kinase for diagnosing Duchenne muscular dystrophy.

Action limits can be set which aid decision-taking, e.g. a cholesterol value in the upper normal range (>6.5 mmol/l) may require therapy.

Patient-specific reference intervals are sometimes required for therapeutic purposes, e.g. specific glucose control criteria for different diabetic patients.

Methods and their normal ranges vary from laboratory to laboratory and according to the sex and age distribution of the reference healthy population. The following results are a general guide for adults' values and may not be apposite for your laboratory.

Haematology

	Male	Female
Haemoglobin	13.5–18.0 g/dl	11.5–16.0 g/dl
Packed cell volume (PCV)	40–54%	37–47%
Red cell count	$4.5–6.5 \times 10^{12}/l$	$3.9–5.6 \times 10^{12}/l$
Mean cell volume (MCV)	76–100 fl	
Mean cell haemoglobin	27–32 pg	
Mean cell haemoglobin concentration	32–36 g/dl	
Reticulocyte count	0.8–2%	
White cell count	$4.0–11.0 \times 10^9/l$	

Platelets	$150–450 \times 10^9/l$	
Prothrombin time	10–14 s	
Activated partial thromboplastin time	30–40 s	
INR therapeutic range for treatment of DVT	2.0–3.0	
Erythrocyte sedimentation rate (ESR)		
Westergren at 1 hour	**Male**	**Female**
	0–10 mm	0–15 mm
	(higher values of ESR may occur in normal elderly patients)	

Cerebrospinal fluid

Cells	0–5 white cells
	0 red cells
Glucose	2.8–4.2 mmol/l
Pressure	70–180 mmH$_2$O
Protein	0.15–0.45 g/l

Clinical chemistry (in SI units)

Serum or plasma

ACE (angiotensin-converting enzyme)	20–54 U/l
Acid phosphatase (total)	1–5 iu/l
Acid phosphatase (prostatic)	0–1 iu/l
ACTH (adrenocorticotrophic hormone)	<80 µg/l
Albumin	35–50 g/l
Aldosterone, recumbent (doubles after 30 min in upright posture)	100–500 pmol/l
Alkaline phosphatase (adult)	80–250 iu/l
Alpha-1 antitrypsin	107–209 mg/dl
Amylase	25–180 Somogyi units/dl
Anion gap	7–16 mmol/l
Aspartate aminotransferase (AST)	15–42 iu/l

Bicarbonate	24–30 mmol/l
Bilirubin (total)	3–17 µmol/l
Bilirubin in babies (toxic value)	>300 µmol/l
Bilirubin (conjugated)	0–5 µmol/l
C-peptide (fasting—interpret with glucose value)	0.2–0.8 nmol/l
C-reactive protein	<10 mg/l
Caeruloplasmin	16–60 mg/dl
Calcitonin	<0.08 µg/l
Calcium (with normal albumin level)	2.12–2.65 mmol/l
Carbon monoxide—non-smoker	0–2%
Carbon monoxide—smoker	up to 5%
Carcinoembryonic antigen (CEA)	0–9 µmol/l
Catecholamines	
– noradrenaline	<5.7 µmol/l
– adrenaline	<2.1 µmol/l
Chloride	95–105 mmol/l
Cholesterol (population reference)	3.9–7.8 mmol/l
Copper	12–26 µmol/l
Cortisol (0900h)	280–700 nmol/l
Cortisol (midnight)	80–280 nmol/l
Creatine kinase (women)	24–195 iu/l
Creatine kinase (men)	24–170 iu/l
Creatinine	70–150 µmol/l
11-Deoxycortisol	7–16 nmol/l
DHEAS (dehydroepiandrosterone sulphate) (women)	4.9–9.4 µmol/l
DHEAS (men)	2.3–12.0 µmol/l
Ferritin (women)	15–140 µg/l
Ferritin (men)	17–230 µg/l
α-Fetoprotein (AFP)	0–14 kU/l
Folate (serum)	2.1–18 µg/l
Folate (red cell)	160–640 µg/l
Follicle-stimulating hormone (female luteal)	2–8 U/l
Follicle-stimulating hormone (postmenopausal women)	>30 U/l

Follicle-stimulating hormone (men)	0.5–5.0 U/l
Gastrin (fasting)	<40 pmol/l
Gastro-inhibitory peptide (fasting)	<300 pmol/l
Glucagon (fasting)	<50 pmol/l
Glucose (plasma, fasting)	3.8–5.5 mmol/l
γ-Glutamyl transpeptidase (women)	7–40 iu/l
γ-Glutamyl transpeptidase (men)	11–51 iu/l
Haemoglobin A_{1c}	4.5–6.2%
HDL (high density lipoprotein) cholesterol	0.8–2.0 mmol/l
Human chorionic gonadotrophin (HCG)	0–5 iu/l
17α-Hydroxyprogesterone	<20 nmol/l
Immunoglobulin A	0.8–3.0 g/l
Immunoglobulin E	<80 kU/l
Immunoglobulin G	6.0–13.0 g/l
Immunoglobulin M	0.4–2.5 g/l
Insulin (fasting — interpret with glucose value)	2–13 mU/l
Iron (women)	11–30 μmol/l
Iron (men)	14–31 μmol/l
Iron-binding capacity	45–70 μmol/l
Lactate (fasting)	0.6–2.0 mmol/l
Lactate dehydrogenase	110–250 iu/l
Lead (blood)	<0.7 μmol/l
Luteinizing hormone (female luteal)	3–6 U/l
Luteinizing hormone (postmenopausal women)	>30 U/l
Luteinizing hormone (men)	3–8 U/l
Magnesium	0.75–1.05 mmol/l
17β-Oestradiol (female luteal)	180–1100 pmol/l
17β-Oestradiol (men)	<220 pmol/l
Osmolality	278–305 mosmol/kg
Parathyroid hormone (PTH)	0.9–5.4 pmol/l
Phosphate	0.8–1.45 mmol/l
Potassium	3.5–5.0 mmol/l
Progesterone (female luteal)	16–77 nmol/l

Progesterone (men)	0–6 nmol/l
Prolactin (women)	<450 mU/l
Prolactin (men)	<400 mU/l
Prostate-specific antigen (PSA)	<4 µg/l
Protein (total)	60–80 g/l
Pyruvate	41–67 µmol/
Renin (recumbent)	1.1–2.7 pmol/ml/h
Renin (erect)	2.8–4.5 pmol/ml/h
Sodium	134–145 mmol/l
Testosterone (women)	1.0–2.5 nmol/l
Testosterone (men)	9–42 nmol/l
Transaminase (GOT, AST)	5–35 iu/l
Transaminase (GPT, ALT)	5–45 iu/l
Triglyceride (fasting)	0.6–1.9 mmol/l
Thyroxine	70–140 nmol/l
Thyroxine (free)	9–25 pmol/l
Triiodothyronine	1.0–3.0 nmol/l
Triiodothyronine (free)	3.4–7.2 pmol/l
TSH (thyroid-stimulating hormone)	0.5–6.0 mU/l
Urate (women)	150–390 µmol/l
Urate (men)	210–480 µmol/l
Urea	2.5–6.7 mmol/l
VIP (vasoactive intestinal polypeptide)	<30 pmol/l
Vitamin B_{12}	150–750 ng/l
Vitamin D	7–50 µg/l
Vitamin E	11.5–35.0 µmol/l
Zinc	6–25 µmol/l

24-hour urine

Aldosterone	10–50 nmol/day
δ-Amino laevulinic acid	9.5–53.4 µmol/day
Calcium	2.5–7.5 mmol/day
Chloride	110–250 mmol/day
Copper	0.2–1.0 µmol/day
Coproporphyrin	51–350 nmol/day
Cortisol	28–280 nmol/day

Creatinine clearance (women)	85–125 ml/min
Creatinine clearance (men)	95–140 ml/min
5-HIAA (5-OH indoleacetic acid)	10.4–41.6 µmol/day
Homovanillic acid (HVA)	<82 µmol/day
Metadrenaline	<2 µmol/day
Normetadrenaline	<3 µmol/day
OH methylmandelic acid (HMMA)	10–35 µmol/day
Osmolality	50–1400 mOsmol/kg
Osmolality (after 12h fluid restriction)	>850 mOsmol/kg
pH	5.5–8.0 pH units
Phosphate	12.9–42 mmol/day
Porphobilinogen	0–10 µmol/day
Potassium	40–120 mmol/day
Protein	50–80 mg/day
Sodium	60–280 mmol/day
Urea	164–600 mmol/day

Drugs in serum

The following are usual therapeutic ranges. The value related to the time of ingestion is crucial for some drugs, e.g. plasma paracetamol >1.0 mmol/l gives a risk of liver damage but the decision interval of the plasma level for therapy decreases with time after an overdose.

Amiodarone—before dose	0.6–2.0 mg/l
Carbamazepine—before dose	34–51 µmol/l
Carbamazepine (children)	17–35 µmol/l
Carbon monoxide—non-smoker	0–2%
Carbon monoxide—smoker	0–5%
Clonazepam—before dose	25–85 µg/l
Digoxin—at least 6 hours after last dose	1.0–2.0 nmol/l
Disopyramide—before dose	2.0–5.0 mg/dl
Epanutin—before dose	40–80 µmol/l
Ethosuximide—before dose	40–80 mg/l
Lithium	0.5–1.5 mmol/l
Phenobarbitone—before dose	65–170 µmol/l
Phenytoin—before dose	40–80 µmol/l

Salicylate	0.4–2.5 mmol/l
Theophylline—before dose	55–110 μmol/l
Valproate—before dose	0.3–0.7 mmol/l

Toxic levels

Barbiturate—potentially fatal	
— short-acting	35 μmol/l
— medium-acting	105 μmol/l
— long-acting	215 μmol/l
Ethanol (physiological <0.2nmol/l)	
— legal limit for driving	<17.4 nmol/l
Paracetamol—risk of liver damage	
— at 4 hours	>1.32 mmol/l
— at 15 hours	<0.2 mmol/l
Salicylate	>2.5 mmol/l

Miscellaneous

| Faecal fat | <18 mmol/day |
| Sweat chloride | 6–40 mmol/l |

Extractable nuclear antigen-binding association

Anti-Ro	SLE, cutaneous lupus
Anti-La	SLE, Sjögren's disease
Anti-Sm	SLE (specific)
Anti-RNP	SLE, mixed connective tissue disease
Anti-Scl-70	Progressive systemic sclerosis
Anti-Jo 1	Polymyositis

CHAPTER 15

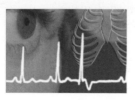

Common Emergency Treatments

Introduction

You will see patients being treated. The following notes provide a guide to the therapies that are employed. In each case a diagnosis needs to be made. The treatments apply to many situations. The specific causes may require additional therapy. These therapies were appropriate in May 2002, but with time other therapies may become more appropriate.

Cardiovascular

Myocardial infarction (classic crushing, central chest pain with radiation to arms, pallor, sweating, distressed ± electrocardiogram (ECG) changes)

- Give 100% oxygen.
- Chew an aspirin — 300 mg.
- Give diamorphine intravenously (i.v.) 2.5–5.0 mg or morphine i.v. 5.0–10.0 mg (± anti-emetic if necessary).
- Attach ECG monitor.
- If ST ≥2 mm new elevation in two or more contiguous chest leads or = 1 mm in standard leads or left bundle-branch block (LBBB):
    - institute thrombolysis with streptokinase, e.g. i.v. 1 500 000 U over 1 hour or tissue plasminogen activator if no contraindication, e.g. bleeding, active peptic ulceration, recent operation, recent cerebral bleed or transient ischaemic attack, aortic aneurysm
    - hydrocortisone i.v. 100 mg if allergic reaction to streptokinase
- If normal blood pressure (BP), well-perfused (warm hands), no heart failure give i.v. β-blocker, e.g. atenolol 5 mg.

- If systolic BP <90 mmHg, periphery cold, monitor central venous pressure (CVP). Consider 200 ml 0.9 g/dl sodium chloride or i.v. dobutamine/adrenaline.
- Treat arrhythmias (NB: do not use lignocaine).
- If left ventricular failure (crepitations, third heart sound, X-ray evidence) give frusemide 40 mg i.v. and consider ACE inhibitors.
- If urine output <30 ml/min, treat as acute renal failure (see below).
- After streptokinase consider s.c. or i.v. heparin.
- If at 24 hours BP >100 mmHg and no heart failure:
  - for oral β-blockers
  - consider oral angiotensin-converting enzyme (ACE) inhibitors if anterior myocardial infarction, previous large myocardial infarction or evidence of heart failure
  - HMG CoA reductase inhibitor
  - Consider antihyperlipidaemic agents.

Unstable angina (continued myocardial pain without evidence of infarction)

- Give 100% oxygen.
- Chew an aspirin (300 mg); buccal GTN.
- Give heparin, e.g. iv. 5000 U bolus followed by infusion 1000 U/h monitor with activated partial thromboplastin time (APTT). Alternatively use low molecular heparin.
- Diamorphine + antiemetic.
- Consider GTN infusion i.v. starting at 1 mg/h, increase up to 10 mg/h as required — keep BP >100 mmHg.
- β-Blocker orally if no clinical evidence of heart failure.
- Calcium antagonist orally, amlodipine if LVF poor or diltiazem if good LVF.
- Consider angioplasty or coronary artery bypass graft (CABG) if pain does not settle (85% will settle on medical treatment).
- Consider antihyperlipidaemic agents.

Acute left ventricular failure (breathless, tachycardia, triple rhythm, crepitations)

- Sit patient up.
- Give 100% oxygen.
- Attach ECG monitor and look for arrhythmias.

- Give i.v. 40–120 mg frusemide or i.v. 1–2 mg bumetanide.
- Give diamorphine i.v. 2.5–5.0 mg or morphine i.v. 5–10 mg (+an antiemetic e.g. i.v. 50 mg cyclizine or prochlorperazine 12.5 mg).
- If ventricular failure persists, consider ACE inhibitor or i.v. nitrate infusion.
- May require continuous positive airway pressure (CPAP) ventilation if no improvement and still dyspnoeic.

Arrhythmia

○ **Bradycardia:** <40 beats/min, light-headed, black-outs, funny turns. Consider atropine 0.6 mg i.v. (repeat to max of 3 mg) or isoprenaline i.v. while waiting for pacemaker.

○ **Tachycardia:** >140 beats/min in compromised patients, e.g. hypotension, heart failure, known heart disease.
  - Narrow-complex:
    - patient shocked: consider DC cardioversion
    - adenosine i.v. 3 mg
      then i.v. 6 mg if necessary
      then i.v. 12 mg if necessary
      then i.v. amiodarone 300 mg in 30 minutes if necessary
    - verapamil i.v. may be used as an alternative (but not with β-blockers)
  - Broad-complex:
    - patient shocked: consider DC cardioversion
    - patient comfortable: lignocane 100 mg i.v. followed by 4 mg/min infusion, reducing as required

○ **Ventricular fibrillation:** see Cardiac arrest instructions (p. 298).

Severe hypertension (e.g. more than 220/120 mmHg,
particularly if symptoms such as headaches or papilloedema)

- Recheck BP, with arterial line and continuous pressure monitoring, if available.
- Bring BP down over 24 hours (rapid reduction contraindicated as can induce cerebral ischaemia).
- Use oral β-blockers, ACE inhibitors or Ca^{2+} channel blocker (but not sublingual nifedipine).

- Or i.v. nitroprusside with arterial monitoring.
- Treat any complications, e.g. left ventricular failure, encephalopathy.

Respiratory

Acute bronchospasm (breathless, wheeze, distress)

- Give 100% oxygen unless known chronic airways disease (see below).
- Ventolin by continuous nebulizer (not inhalers) 5 ml in 2 ml water.
- Hydrocortisone 100 mg i.v. or oral prednisolone 30–50 mg.
- Aminophylline 5 mg/kg i.v. by slow injection (10–15 minutes) but **not** if patient has been taken theophyllines already.
- Do blood gases:

	Po_2 (in pKa)	Pco_2 (in pKa)
— Mild	<10	<4
— Moderate	8–10	<4
— Severe	<8	4–6: watch carefully
— Desperate	<7	>6: consider ventilation

- Monitor fatigue—consider ventilation if patient becomes exhausted.

Acute exacerbation in chronic obstructive airways disease (usually breathless, cough, sputum and coarse crepitations)

- Give 24% oxygen and increase if Pco_2 not raised.
- Blood gases:
  - $Po_2\downarrow$ and $Pco_2\downarrow$ 'pink puffer': increase oxygen content
  - $Po_2\downarrow$ and $Pco_2\uparrow$ 'blue bloater': increase oxygen carefully, repeating blood gases, as removal of hypoxic drive may decrease respiratory volume and rate. Then reduce Po_2 and consider doxapram. Ventilation may be indicated when there is a good prognosis
- Physiotherapy to cough up sputum.
- Culture sputum, chest X-ray, consider antibiotics.

Gastrointestinal

Acute gastrointestinal haemorrhage (sudden
collapse, haematemasis or red/black sticky stools; BP <100 mmHg,
pulse >100 beats/min)

- Assess whether cirrhosis/portal hypertension, peptic ulcer.
- i.v. access (2 large venflons) and take blood for haematology,
  biochemistry and crossmatching.
- If BP <90 mmHg, 500 ml 0.9 g/dl sodium chloride or colloid in 30
  minutes.
- If no BP, consider group 0 rhesus-negative blood.
- If no central pulse, for cardiorespiratory resuscitation.
- Monitor CVP.
- Give blood as required to raise BP and CVP.
- Urinary catheter if severe blood loss.
- Alert surgical team and arrange urgent endoscopy.

Acute hepatic failure (jaundice, foetor, liver flap,
confusion)

- If systolic BP <90 mmHg, 500 ml i.v. 5% dextrose or colloid in 30
  minutes.
- Monitor CVP.
- Monitor blood glucose—if <4 mmol/l, infuse dextrose 10% and
  recheck.
- Look for drugs, including paracetamol overdose.
- Look for infection—blood, chest, urine, ascites.
    - Look for occult bleeding, including increasing plasma urea:
- consider fresh frozen plasma to correct clotting
- Start oral lactulose, consider neomycin.
- Prevent stress ulcers with H_2-blocker or proton pump blocker.
- Vitamins B and K i.v.
- Restrict salt and water intake.
- Monitor drugs, electrolyte, liver function tests, clotting, pH.

Neurological

Epileptic attack (tonic/clonic movements, usually unconscious)

- Oxygen.
- Diazepam i.v. 5–10 mg over 2 minutes, then i.v. 2 mg/min for 20 minutes or until fit ceases. Watch for respiratory depression.
- Bedside test for glucose — ?hypoglycaemia.
- Phenytoin i.v. 50 mg/min.
- If fit continues:
    - chlormethiazole or phenytoin
    - general anaesthesia and ventilate

Unconsciousness with no overt cause

- Clear airway and give 100% oxygen.
- Prone recovery position unless airway protected by endotracheal tube.
- Examine for head injury, neurological deficit, neck stiffness.
- Enquire whether diabetic or access to insulin, any tablets or whether a suicide risk.
- Prevent fitting (see above).
- If respiratory rate <10 breaths/min give i.v. naloxone.
- Check blood glucose.
- If BP <90 mmHg systolic, give 500 ml 0.9 g/dl sodium chloride or colloid i.v.
- Check blood gases.
- Take blood and urine for drug tests.
- Document level of consciousness on Glasgow Coma Scale.

Meningitis (headache, neck stiffness, vomiting, photophobia, febrile)

- **N.B.** if purpuric rash immediately start i.v. antibiotic — ceftriaxone 2 g — after taking blood cultures.
- Check for signs of raised intracranial pressure, e.g. papilloedema.
- Lumbar puncture if no signs of raised intracranial pressure:
    - note pressure

- cerebrospinal fluid (CSF) for culture — bacterial, PCR for viruses, biochemistry and microscopy
- Cloudy CSF (white cells) — prompt i.v. antibiotics after blood cultures.
- Blood-stained — assess whether bloody tap, i.e. blood at first then clearing, or subarachnoid haemorrhage (consistent blood with xanthochromia of CSF after centrifuging down red cells).

Other systems

Acute renal failure (rapid increase in plasma creatinine, urine output <30 ml/h)

- Consider **prerenal** cause (patient 'dehydrated' — dry tongue, low skin turgor, empty veins, low CVP, low blood pressure) — give fluid challenge and continue until JVP is 2–3 cm above the manubriosternal junction.
- Consider **postrenal** cause (e.g. enlarged prostate, bilateral ureteric stones, renal/pelviureteric obstruction). If large prostate and large bladder, consider passing catheter.
- If no obvious cause of renal failure, ultrasound abdomen — ?dilated ureters or dilated renal pelves or small kidneys, indicating chronic renal failure.
- Check plasma potassium, sodium, creatinine, urea (if potassium >6 mmol/l and ECG changes, give i.v. glucose/insulin, i.v. calcium gluconate and rectal cation exchange resin).
- Check urine sodium and osmolality
    - in prerenal failure, urine osmolality >400 mosmol/kg and sodium <30 mmol/l
    - in renal failure, <400 mosmol/kg and >30 mmol/l, respectively
- Microscope urine sediment for red cells, white cells, casts and bacteria.
- Check arterial pH.
- If incipient renal tubular necrosis, for i.v. frusemide 80–500 mg.
- When fluid-replete, restrict fluid to 500 ml per day + previous day's losses.

- High-energy, low-protein diet.
- Watch for infection.
- Consider dialysis if creatinine >400 μmol/l or potassium remains >6 mmol/l, fluid overload, acidosis or pericarditis.

Diabetic ketoacidosis (usually known diabetic patient; ketoacidosis induced by infection, vomiting, missing insulin injections; patient is drowsy, 'dehydrated' ± ketotic breath)

- Check plasma glucose, electrolytes, arterial pH, CRP, troponin, blood and urine culture, ECG and CXR.
- Check urine for ketones; measure in ketone meter if possible, otherwise use serum or urinary ketones. If there are no ketones consider hyperosmolar, non-ketotic coma.
- Fluid replacement—initially N saline—typically 1 l over 30 mins, 1 l over 2 h, 1 l over 4 h, 1 l over 6 h then 8-hourly. When glucose levels are less than 11 mmol/l switch to 5% dextrose. (Remember this would need to be modified with co-morbidity, e.g. CCF.)
  - CVP line to assess volume requirement may be necessary
- Stat dose of insulin 10 units actrapid IM.
- Insulin infusion (50 units actrapid in 50 ml of N saline to run i.v. according to sliding scale): aim to reduce glucose level by 6 mmol/h. sliding scale:

Glucose (mmol/l)	Insulin (U/hour)
>20	6
17–20	5
14–17	4
11–14	3
7–10	2
4–7	1
<4	0.5

- Measure ketones and glucose hourly and adjust insulin accordingly.
- If very drowsy, nasogastric tube to prevent inhalation of vomit.
- Potassium replacement—none if K^+ <5.5 mmol/l. Otherwise, add potassium 20–40 mmol/l to each litre of i.v. saline.

Hypoglycaemia (symptoms include drowsy/unconscious, perspiring, tachycardia, bounding pulse, usually in insulin-treated diabetic due to missing snack or increased exercise. N.B. many diabetic patients are asymptomatic with hypoglycaemia)
- Check plasma glucose. (Do not await result from laboratory — treat straight away.)
- Keep airway clear.
- If no i.v. access give 1 mg glucagon i.m., acts in 5–10 minutes (but not if hypoglycaemia due to insulinoma).
- If emergency, e.g. fitting, 50 ml 50 g/dl i.v. glucose followed by 50 ml of 0.9 g/dl saline to wash sclerosant, hypertonic glucose out of vein.

Septicaemia (febrile >39°C, rigors)
- Give 100% oxygen.
- Look for source of septicaemia.
- If systolic BP <90 mmHg, 500 ml i.v. sodium chloride or colloid i.v. in 30 minutes.
- Monitor CVP.
- Antibiotics i.v. after blood cultures, culture of urine, throat or pustules.
- If BP ↓, pH ↓ or consciousness level ↓ — transfer to intensive care unit.

Poisoning or overdose
- Give 100% oxygen, except in paraquat poisoning.
- Check paracetamol and aspirin levels in all patients.
- Give naloxone if respiratory rate <10 breaths/min. Measure blood gases and consider ventilation.
- Correct hypotension: if BP <90 mmHg, 500 ml i.v. sodium chloride in 30 minutes.
- Consider gastric lavage — intubate first if unconscious.
- Paracetamol overdose — acetylcysteine according to blood levels of paracetamol.
- Aspirin overdose:
  - gastric lavage up to 12 hours
  - watch pH

- consider forced alkaline diuresis
- Amphetamine poisoning:
  - beware sudden airway oedema
  - have available intubation equipment, adrenaline, chlorpheniramine, hydrocortisone
- Consider activated charcoal per oral/gastric tube.
- If potentially an unusual poison, phone poison centre for advice.

Anaphylactic response

- Give 100% oxygen.
- Chlorpheniramine 10 mg i.v. in 1 minute.
- Hydrocortisone 100 mg i.v.
- If severe, adrenaline 0.5–1 mg i.v. slowly over 1–2 minutes.
- If BP <90 mmHg, 500 ml i.v. sodium chloride or colloid.

Death

Whilst diagnosis of death *per se* does not require emergency therapy, the required procedures are an important aspect of medicine.

If there is sudden loss of consciousness, consider cardiopulmonary resuscitation—see Cardiac arrest instructions (p. 298).

- Pale, pulseless, apnoeic—listen at mouth, observe chest.
- No heart sounds—listen with diaphragm.
- Fixed pupils.
- Head and eyes move together when head moved, i.e. no oculocephalic reflex movement or 'doll's eye' movement.
- No corneal response.
- No response to any stimulus.

If patient cold, <35°C, or major drug overdose, e.g. barbiturate, patients can appear dead. If in doubt look at retina with ophthalmoscope to see if 'trucking' of non-flowing segments of blood in veins.

Brain death criteria

- If the patient is on a ventilator because of apnoea, test:
  - at least 6 hours after onset of coma
  - at least 24 hours after cardiac arrest/circulation restoration

- by two independent consultants if feasible
- Whether patient has condition that could lead to irremediable brain damage.
- There are no reflex responses or epileptic jerks.
- No hypothermia — temperature >35°C.
- No drug intoxication — off therapy for 48 hours
    - particularly depressants, neuromuscular-blocking (relaxant) drugs
- No hypoglycaemia, acidosis, gross electrolyte imbalance.
- All brainstem reflexes absent, confirmed by two physicians:
    - no pupil response to light
- no corneal reflexes
- no vestibular-ocular reflexes:
    - visualize tympanic membranes
    - 20 ml cold water in each ear
    - no eye movements
- no cranial motor responses:
    - no gag reflex
    - no cough reflex to bronchial stimulaton
- no respiratory effort when ventilator is stopped:
    - P_{CO_2} rise to 6.7 kPa
- Repeat tests at least 2 hours later, usually after 24 hours.
- Time of second test is legally the time of death.

N.B. Spinal reflexes and electroencephalogram are irrelevant. Warn family that reflex leg movements can exist after cessation of brainstem function and are not of relevance.

Appendices

Appendix 1: Jaeger reading chart

Jaeger types assess visual acuity for close tasks. It provides the easiest quick method of assessment. The patient should use his spectacles normally required for reading. Ask the patient to read the smallest type he can read, if read with few mistakes, ask him to read the next size down. Record the size of type that can be read with each eye separately.

Hope, they say, deserts us at no period of our existence. From first to last, and in the face of smarting disillusions we continue to expect good fortune, better health, and better conduct; and that so confidently, that we judge it needless to deserve them. I think it improbable that I shall ever write like Shakespeare, conduct an army like Hannibal, or distinguish

Here we recognise the thoughts of our boyhood; and our boyhood ceased — well, when? — not, I think, at twenty; nor, perhaps, altogether at twenty-five: nor yet at thirty: and possibly to be quite frank, we are still in the thick of that arcadian period. For as the race of man, after centuries of civilisation, still keeps

I have always suspected public taste to be a mongrel product, out of affectation by dogmatism; and felt sure, if you could only find an honest man of no special literary bent, he would tell you he thought much of Shakespeare bombastic and most absurd, and all of him written in very

If you look back on your own education, I am sure it will not be the full, vivid, instructive hours of truancy that you regret: and you would rather cancel some lack-lustre period between sleep and waking in the class. For my own part, I have attended

There is a sort of dead-alive, hackneyed people about, who are scarcely conscious of living except in the exercise of some conventional occupation.

Books are good enough in their own way, but they are a mighty bloodless substitute for life. It seems a pity to sit, like the Lady of Shalott, peering into a mirror,

The other day, a ragged, barefoot boy ran down the street after a marble, with so jolly an air that he set every one he passed

A happy man or woman is a better thing to find than a

"How now, young fellow, what dost thou

"Truly, sir, I

Appendix 2: Visual acuity 3m chart

The 3-m Snellen chart should be held at 3m from the patient, with good lighting, with each of the patient's eyes covered in turn. Use the patient's usual spectacles for this distance. If the patient cannot read 6/6 (e.g. 6/12 is best vision in one eye), repeat without spectacles and with a 'pinhole' that largely nullifies refractive errors. Note for each eye the best acuity obtained and the method used, e.g. L 6/9 R 6/6 with spectacles.

V H

36

XUA

24

HTYO

18

VUAXT

12

HAYOUX

9

YUXTHAOV

6

XOATVHUY

5

Appendix 3: Hodkinson ten point mental test score

A simple test of impaired cognitive function (see p. 156).

1 Age	must be correct
2 Time	without looking at clock or watch, and correct to nearest hour
3 42 West Street	give this (or similar) address twice, ask patient to repeat immediately (to check it has registered), and test recall at end of procedure
4 Recognize two people	point at nurse and other, ask: '*Who is that person? what does she/he do?*'
5 Year	exact, except in January when previous year is accepted
6 Name of place	may ask type of place, or area of town
7 Date of birth	exact
8 Start of World War 1	exact year
9 Name of present monarch	
10 Count from 20 to 1	backwards, may prompt with 20/19/18, no other prompts; patient may hesitate and self-correct but no other errors (tests concentration)

Check recall of address (question 3 above)

Total score out of 10

Communication problems (e.g. *deafness*, *dysphasia*) or abnormal mood (e.g. *depression*) may affect the mental test score, and should be noted. (After Qureshi, K. & Hodkinson, H. Evaluation of a ten-question mental test in the institutional elderly. *Age Ageing* 1974;**3**:152.)

Appendix 4: Barthel index of activities of daily living

An assessment of disabilities affecting key functions that influence a person's mobility, self-care and independence (see p. 157).

Bowels:
  0 = incontinent (or needs to be given enema)
  1 = occasional accident (once per week or less)
  2 = continent (for preceding week)

Bladder:
  0 = incontinent or catheterized and unable to manage alone
  1 = occasional accident (once per day or less)
  2 = continent (for preceding week)

Feeding:
  0 = unable
  1 = needs help cutting, spreading butter, etc.
  2 = independent

Grooming:
  0 = needs help with personal care
  1 = independent face/hair/teeth/shaving (implements provided)

Dressing:
  0 = dependent
  1 = needs help but can do about half unaided
  2 = independent (including buttons, zips, laces, etc.)

Transfer bed to chair and back:
  0 = unable, no sitting balance
  1 = major help (one strong/skilled or two people), can sit up
  2 = minor help from one person (physical or verbal)
  3 = independent

Toilet use:
  0 = dependent
  1 = needs some help, but can do something alone
  2 = independent (on and off, dressing, wiping)

Mobility around house or ward, indoors:
  0 = immobile
  1 = wheelchair independent, including corners

2 = walks with help of one person (physical, verbal, supervision)

3 = independent (but may use any aid, e.g. stick)

Stairs:

0 = unable

1 = needs help (physical, verbal, carrying aid)

2 = independent

Bathing:

0 = dependent

1 = independent (in and out of bath or shower)

Total score out of 20

Guidelines for the Barthel index of activities of daily living (ADL):

1 The index should be used as a record of what a patient does, not what a patient *can* do.

2 The main aim is to establish the degree of independence from any help, physical or verbal, however minor and for whatever reason.

3 The need for supervision renders the patient not independent.

4 A patient's performance should be established using the best available evidence. The patient, friends/relatives and nurses are the usual sources, but direct observation and common sense are also important. Direct testing is not necessary.

5 Usually the patient's performance over the preceding 24–48 hours is important, but occasionally longer periods will be relevant.

6 Middle categories imply that the patient supplies over 50% of the effort.

7 The use of aids to be independent is allowed.

(After Collin, C., Wade, D.T., Davies, S. & Horne, V. The Barthel ADL index: a reliability study. *Int Disabil Studies* 1988;**10**:61–63.)

Appendix 5: Cardiac arrest instructions

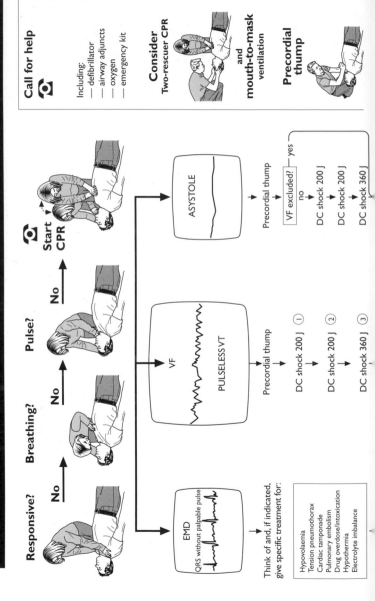

Responsive? No → **Breathing?** No → **Pulse?** No → **Start CPR**

Call for help

Including:
— defibrillator
— airway adjuncts
— oxygen
— emergency kit

Consider
Two-rescuer CPR
and
mouth-to-mask ventilation

Precordial thump

EMD
QRS without palpable pulse

Think of and, if indicated, give specific treatment for:

Hypovolaemia
Tension pneumothorax
Cardiac tamponade
Pulmonary embolism
Drug overdose/intoxication
Hypothermia
Electrolyte imbalance

VF
PULSELESS VT

Precordial thump

DC shock 200 J ①
DC shock 200 J ②
DC shock 360 J ③

ASYSTOLE

Precordial thump

VF excluded? — yes
no
DC shock 200 J
DC shock 200 J
DC shock 360 J

Place paddles

If flat trace, check switches, connections and gain

Give oxygen

Intubate

Cannulate large vein

Continue CPR

If not already
· intubate
· i.v. access

↓

Adrenaline 1 mg i.v.

↓

10 CPR sequences of
1:5 ventilation/compression

If not already
· intubate
· i.v. access

↓

Adrenaline 1 mg i.v.

↓

10 CPR sequences of
1:5 ventilation/compression

↓

DC shock 360 J ④

DC shock 360 J ⑤

DC shock 360 J ⑥

If not already
· intubate
· i.v. access

↓

Adrenaline 1 mg i.v.

↓

10 CPR sequences of
1:5 ventilation/compression

(Atropine 3 mg i.v. once only)

Electrical activity evident?

no → yes → Pace

If no response after three cycles, consider high dose adrenaline 5 mg i.v.

Consider
· pressor agent
· calcium
· alkalizing agents
· adrenaline 5 mg i.v.

1 The interval between shocks 3 and 4 should not be > 2 min
2 Adrenaline given during loop approx. every 2–3 min
3 Continue loops for as long as defibrillation is indicated
4 After three loops consider · alkalizing agents
                                · antiarrhythmic agents

POST-RESUSCITATION CARE
Check
· arterial blood gases
· electrolytes
· chest X-ray
Observe monitor and treat patient in an intensive care area

If an i.v. line cannot be established, consider giving double or triple doses of adrenaline or atropine via an endotracheal tube

PROLONGED RESUSCITATION:
consider alkalizing agents, e.g. 50 mmol sodium bicarbonate (50 ml of 8.4%) or according to blood gas results

Index

Note: page numbers in *italics* refer to figures, those in **bold** refer to tables. Plates are referred to by Plate number and are located between pages 150 and 151

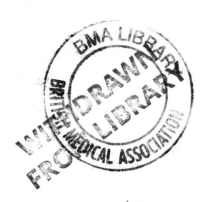